100 No-Equipment Workouts
Volume 2
2017

N. Rey | darebee.com

Printed in the United Kingdom. First Printing, 2016

ISBN 13: 978-1-84481-005-5
ISBN 10: 1-84481-005-4

Warning and Disclaimer
Although every precaution has been taken to verify the accuracy of the information contained herein, the author and publisher assume no responsibility for any errors or omissions. No liability is assumed for damage or injury that may result from the use of information contained within.

Fitness is a journey, not a destination.
Darebee, Project

100 workouts - Volume II

1. 2-Minute Abs
2. Abs Upgrade
3. Altered Carbon
4. Armory
5. Banshee
6. Bat Out of Hell
7. BBQ Workout
8. Berserker
9. Big Bang
10. Body Mod
11. Body Patch
12. Bootcamp
13. Bottom Line
14. Bounty Hunter
15. Boxer Abs
16. Boxer Flexibility
17. Boxer Power
18. Cardio Combat
19. Cardio Demon
20. Cardio Drill
21. Cardio Fire
22. Cardio Light
23. Cardio Melt
24. Cardio Sofa
25. Caterpillar-Butterfly
26. Centurion
27. Cerberus
28. Chapter One
29. Chase
30. Chimera
31. Chisel
32. Code Zero
33. Commander
34. Commando
35. Conqueror
36. Cossack
37. Crusher
38. Cypher
39. Damage Control
40. Danger Zone
41. Deadlock
42. Death by Burpees
43. Demolition
44. Dirty 30
45. Double Dash
46. Ender
47. Express Abs
48. Finisher
49. Finish Line
50. Free Fall
51. Fullbody Render
52. Gambit
53. Heist
54. Hell Diver
55. Hell Raider
56. Hightail
57. Hunter
58. Huntsman
59. Inferno
60. Initiation
61. Iron Bar
62. Iron Claw
63. Iron Fist
64. Iron Maiden
65. Kamikaze
66. King of the Hill
67. Kitsune
68. Knockout
69. Kraken
70. Launch Codes
71. Live Wire
72. Lumberjack
73. Mutiny
74. Night Shift
75. No Capes
76. Off the Grid
77. One Punch
78. Part 2
79. Plan B
80. Power Mode
81. Power Run
82. P.S.
83. Punch Out
84. Push-Up Massacre
85. Ragnarok
86. Reboot
87. Recon Squad
88. Recruit
89. Scorcher
90. Sculptor
91. Sentinel
92. Sniper
93. Splits
94. Springboard
95. Static Zap
96. Superplank
97. Tank Top
98. Top to Bottom
99. Valkyrie
100. Watch Me

Introduction

Bodyweight training may look easy, but if you are not used to it, it's very far from that. It is just as intense as running and it is just as challenging so if you struggle with it at the very beginning, it's perfectly ok – you will get better at it once you start doing it regularly. Do it at your own pace and take longer breaks if you need to.

You can start with a single individual workout from the collection and see how you feel. If you are new to bodyweight training always start any workout on Level I (level of difficulty).

You can pick any number of workouts per week, usually between 3 and 5 and rotate them for maximum results.

Some workouts are more suitable for weight loss and toning up and others are more strength oriented, some do both. To make it easier for you to choose, they have all been labelled according to FOCUS, use it to design a training regimen based on your goal.

High Burn and Strength oriented workouts will help you with your weight, aerobic capacity and muscle tone, some are just more specialized, but it doesn't mean you should exclusively focus on one or the other. Whatever your goal with bodyweight training you'll benefit from doing exercises that produce results in both areas.

This collection has been designed to be completely no-equipment for maximum accessibility so several bodyweight exercises like pull-ups have been excluded. If you want to work on your biceps and back more and you have access to a pull-up bar, have one at home or can use it somewhere else like the nearest playground (monkey bars), you can do wide and close grip pull-ups, 3 sets to failure 2-3 times a week with up to 2 minutes rest in between sets in addition to your training. Alternatively, you can add pull-ups at the beginning or at the end of every set of a Strength Oriented workout.

All of the routines in this collection are suitable for both men and women, no age restrictions apply.

The Manual

Workout posters are read from left to right and contain the following information: grid with exercises (images), number of reps (repetitions) next to each, number of sets for your fitness level (I, II or III) and rest time.

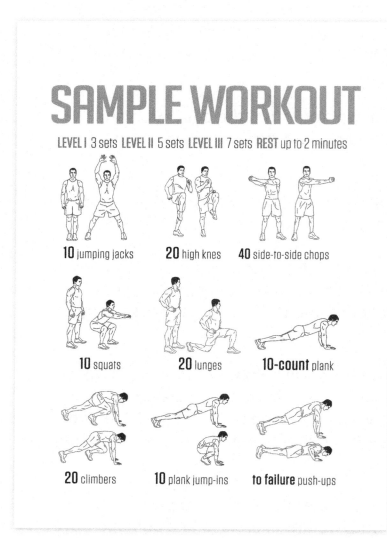

Difficulty Levels:

Level I: normal
Level II: hard
Level III: advanced

1 set

10 jumping jacks
20 high knees (10 each leg)
40 side-to-side chops (20 each side)
10 squats
20 lunges (10 each leg)
10-count plank (hold while counting to 10)
20 climbers (10 each leg)
10 plank jump-ins
to failure push-ups (your maximum)

Up to 2 minutes rest between sets

30 seconds, 60 seconds or 2 minutes - it's up to you.

"Reps" stands for repetitions, how many times an exercise is performed. Reps are usually located next to each exercise's name. Number of reps is always a total number for both legs / arms / sides. It's easier to count this way: e.g. if it says 20 climbers, it means that both legs are already counted in - it is 10 reps each leg.

Reps to failure means to muscle failure = your personal maximum, you repeat the move until you can't. It can be anything from one rep to twenty, normally applies to more challenging exercises. The goal is to do as many as you possibly can.

The transition from exercise to exercise is an important part of each circuit (set) - it is often what makes a particular workout more effective. Transitions are carefully worked out to hyperload specific muscle groups more for better results. For example if you see a plank followed by push-ups it means that you start performing push-ups right after you finished with the plank avoiding dropping your body on the floor in between.

There is no rest between exercises - only after sets, unless specified otherwise. You have to complete the entire set going from one exercise to the next as fast as you can before you can rest.

What does "up to 2 minutes rest" mean: it means you can rest for up to 2 minutes but the sooner you can go again the better. Eventually your recovery time will improve naturally, you won't need all two minutes to recover - and that will also be an indication of your improving fitness.

Recommended rest time:

Level I: 2 minutes or less
Level II: 60 seconds or less
Level III: 30 seconds or less

If you can't do all out push-ups yet on Level I it is perfectly acceptable to do knee push-ups instead. The modification works the same muscles as a full push-up but lowers the load significantly helping you build up on it first. It is also ok to switch to knee push-ups at any point if you can no longer do full push-ups in the following sets.

Video Exercise Library
http://darebee.com/exercises

The workouts are organized in alphabetical order so you can find the workouts you favor easier and faster.

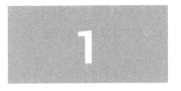

2-Minute Abs

If you only have two minutes to spare towards some exercise you can do no better than the 2-Minute Abs workout. Abs are required every time we do something physical and they play a pivotal role in supporting the spine, affecting posture and enhancing physical performance. The 2-Minute Abs program helps you strengthen this critically important muscle group.

Focus: Abs

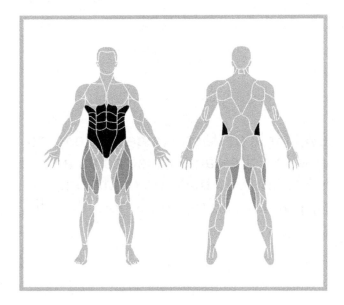

2-minute abs

DAREBEE WORKOUT © darebee.com

20 seconds each exercise | no rest between exercises

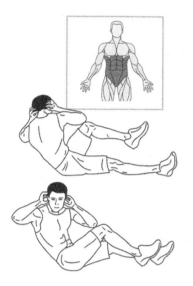

1. knee-to-elbow crunches

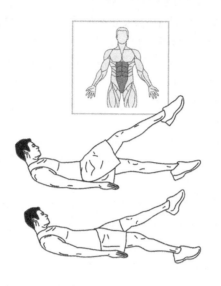

2. flutter kicks

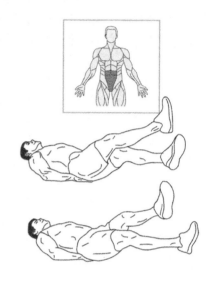

3. scissors

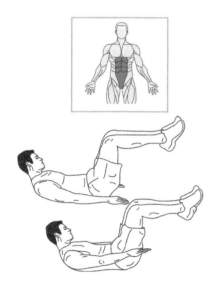

4. hundreds

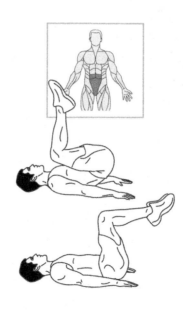

5. reverse crunches

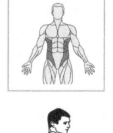
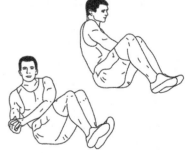

6. sitting twists

2   Abs Upgrade

Abs are not just the engine that powers some of your most energetic movements, they also play a vital role in protecting a vulnerable part of your body. The Abs Upgrade workout works each of the four major abdominal muscle groups for that all-in feeling.

Focus: Abs

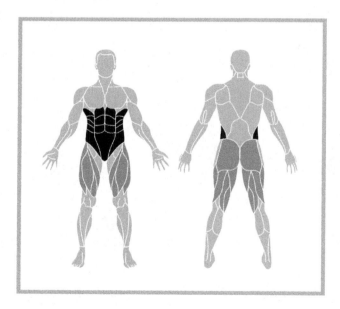

abs upgrade

DAREBEE WORKOUT © darebee.com

LEVEL I 3 sets **LEVEL II** 4 sets **LEVEL III** 5 sets **REST** up to 2 minutes

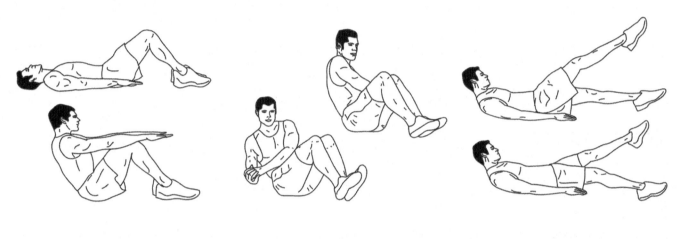

20 sit-ups   **20** sitting twists   **20** flutter kicks

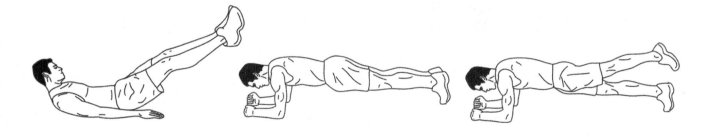

20-count raised leg hold   **20-count** plank   **20-count** raised leg plank

3   Altered Carbon

Exercise is designed to allow us to do one thing in particular: be the best version of ourselves we can be. The Altered Carbon workout is (with a knowing reference to a popular sci-fi book) designed to help you improve yourself, augment your capabilities and become ...well, a new improved model of you.

Focus: High Burn

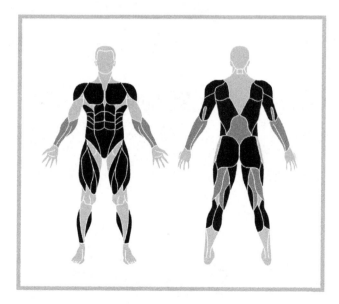

ALTERED CARBON

DAREBEE WORKOUT
© darebee.com
LEVEL I 3 sets
LEVEL II 5 sets
LEVEL III 7 sets
REST up to 2 minutes

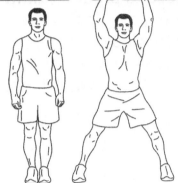

10 jumping jacks

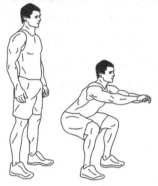

10 squats

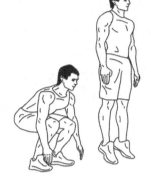

5 jump squats

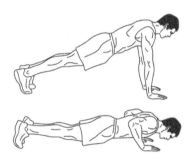

10 push-ups

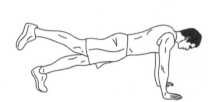

10-count raised leg hold

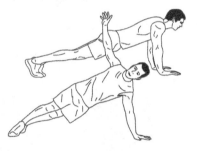

10 plank rotations

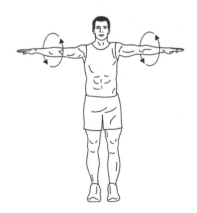

10 raised arm rotations

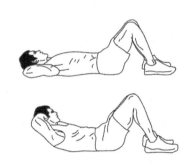

10 crunches

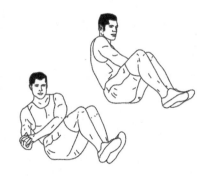

10 sitting twists

4 Armory

Armory is a full body workout that targets fascial fitness to produce extra power and explosiveness in every move you make. The moves are designed to force muscles to work in a precise way through upper body combat moves and as fatigue begins to kick in, you find yourself in the sweat zone, using your entire body as a primary weapon. Do it with EC and you will also fill the burn faster.

Focus: Strength & Tone

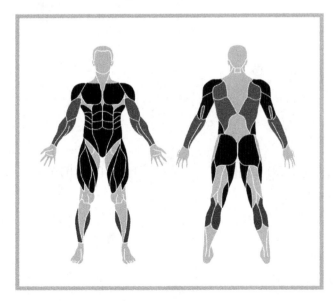

ARMORY

DAREBEE WORKOUT © darebee.com

LEVEL I 3 sets **LEVEL II** 5 sets **LEVEL III** 7 sets **REST** up to 2 minutes

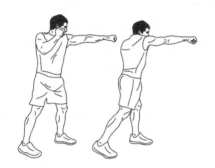

60 punches

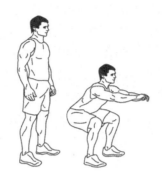

10 squats

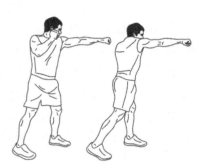

60 punches

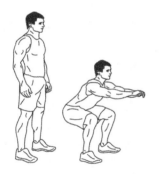

10 squats

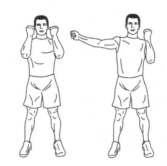

60 side-to-side backfists

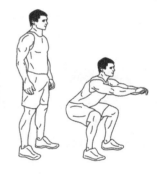

10 squats

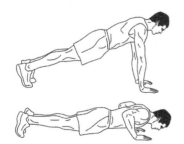

10 push-ups

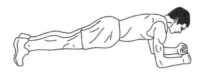

30-count elbow plank

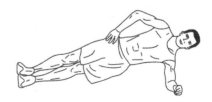

30-count side plank

5 Banshee

When it's just you against the world and the only clue you have is that the odds are stacked against you, you know that the only way you can survive is by hankering down and working the basics. A strong core, legs that you can command and arms that can piston out punches are the assets in your toolbox. Now all you have to do is face impossible odds, take on an endless array of opponents in sequential order and hope that the love of your life finds her way back to you. We can't promise anything here beyond you building good core strength, agility, body control and a strong belief in yourself. Now go and get them and should you find yourself on a side of the law you just never expected to be, just roll with it.

Focus: Strength & Tone

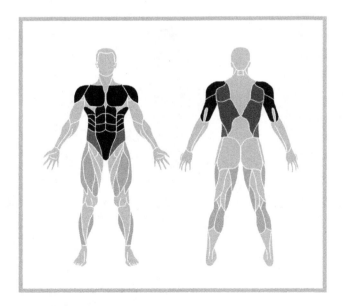

BANSHEE

DAREBEE WORKOUT © darebee.com

LEVEL I 3 sets **LEVEL II** 4 sets **LEVEL III** 5 sets **REST** up to 2 minutes

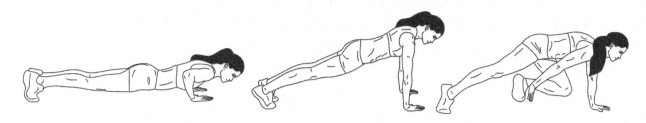

10combos push-up + climber tap (each foot)

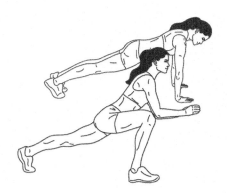 **10** plank into lunges

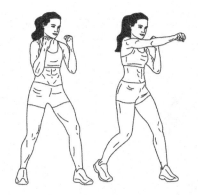 **40** punches

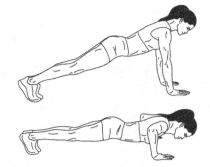 **10** wide grip push-ups

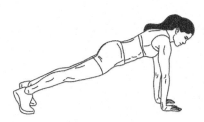
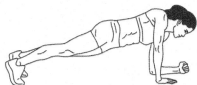
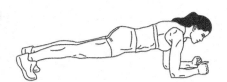

10 up and down planks

6   Bat Out of Hell

Bat Out Of Hell is a quick, pacey workout that delivers a high burn through just three exercises. The alternating load on the muscles as you go from one to the other ensures that you get to recover on the fly as muscles are alternatively used in a concentric and eccentric way. Go for EC for that extra burn deep in your lungs and you know that you are doing it right.

Focus: High Burn

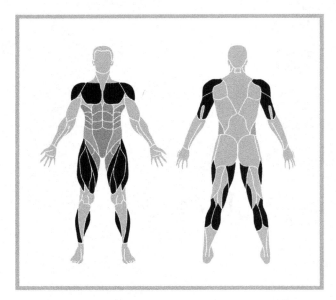

BAT OUT OF HELL

DAREBEE WORKOUT © darebee.com
LEVEL I 3 sets **LEVEL II** 5 sets **LEVEL III** 7 sets
2 minutes rest between sets

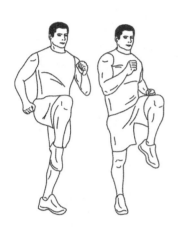
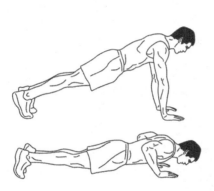
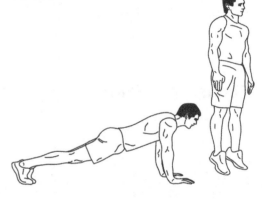

40 high knees

4 push-ups

40 high knees

4 basic burpees w/ jump

40 high knees

4 push-ups

40 high knees

4 basic burpees w/ jump

done

7   BBQ Workout

When you're ready to move your chops, cook your goose and face some high stakes, you're ready for our BBQ workout. When all the cliche references are left behind you're left with a workout that will really put your body through the motions until you really feel cooked.

Focus: High Burn

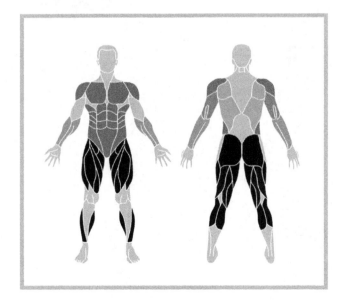

BBQ

DAREBEE WORKOUT
© darebee.com
LEVEL I 3 sets
LEVEL II 5 sets
LEVEL III 7 sets
REST up to 2 minutes

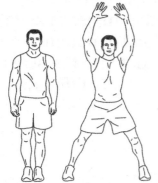

20 jumping jacks

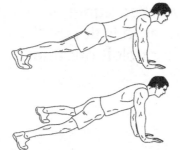

4 plank jacks

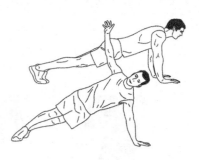

20 jumping jacks

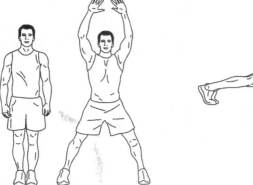

4 climbers

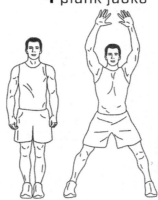

20 jumping jacks

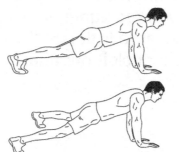

4 plank rotations

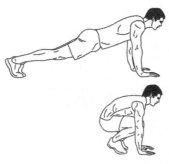

20 jumping jacks

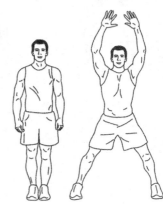

4 plank jump-ins

20 jumping jacks

8 Berserker

Some body-strength orientated workouts are designed to kick your butt and Berserker is one of them. From one exercise to another major muscle groups are worked and then worked again but with the load constantly changing there is time to recover (a little) on the fly. You get into the sweat zone form the very first set but stick it out and you will feel the difference when you finish.

Focus: Strength & Tone

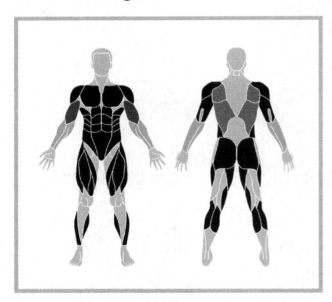

BERSERKER

LEVEL I 3 sets **LEVEL II** 5 sets **LEVEL III** 7 set **REST** up to 2 minutes

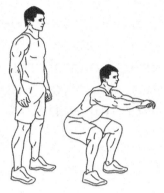

20 squats

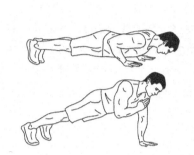

10 push-up + shoulder tap

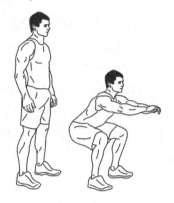

20 squats

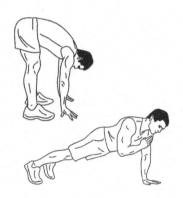

10 walk-out + shoulder tap

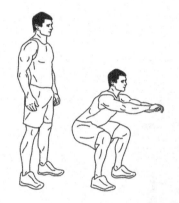

20 squats

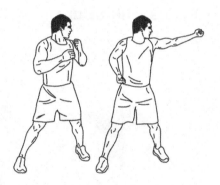

20 backfists

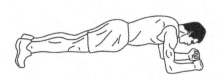

20sec elbow plank

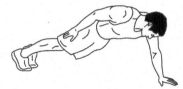

20sec one arm plank

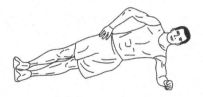

20sec side plank

9 Big Bang

A fast, energetic, cardio-pumping workout helps work up a good sweat, get your body moving and burn up some calories. The Big Bang workout does all of that but in addition its switch from speed to strength also challenges the muscle control you have over your body. This is perfect when you want to exercise but are not sure what you want to do but still do not want to feel cheated out of a good work out.

Focus: High Burn

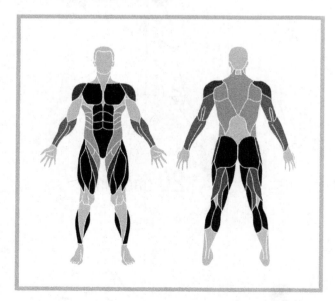

BIG BANG

DAREBEE WORKOUT
© darebee.com
LEVEL I 3 sets
LEVEL II 5 sets
LEVEL III 7 sets
REST up to 2 minutes

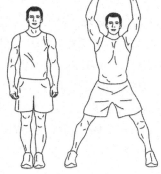
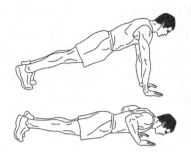
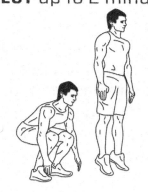

10 jumping jacks   **5** push-ups   **5** jump squats

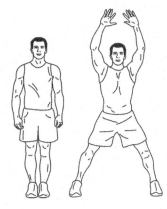
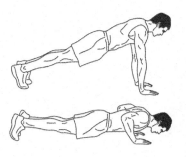
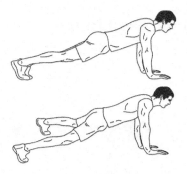

10 jumping jacks   **5** push-ups   **5** plank jacks

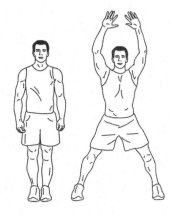
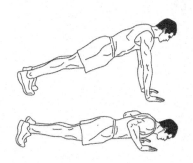
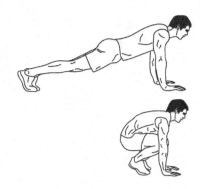

10 jumping jacks   **5** push-ups   **5** plank jump-ins

10   Body Mod

If you are looking for a full-body workout that will get you into the sweat zone fast and help you build up speed, endurance and overall body strength then Body Mod is exactly what you need. Bring your knees to waist height when doing both March Steps and High Knees, go for height on Jump Squats and reduce rest between sets to EC levels and what you have is a powerful weapon you can use to unlock the potential of your own physical abilities.

Focus: High Burn

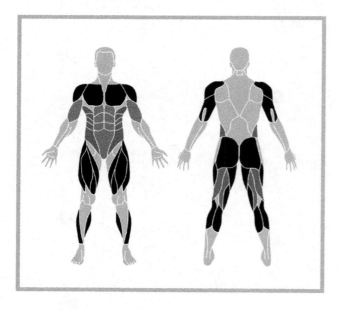

BODY MOD

DAREBEE WORKOUT © darebee.com

LEVEL I 3 sets **LEVEL II** 5 sets **LEVEL III** 7 sets **REST** up to 2 minutes

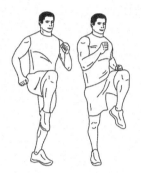

20 high knees

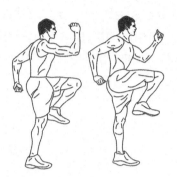

20 march steps

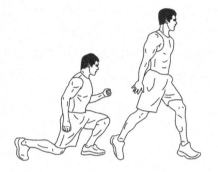

10 jumping lunges

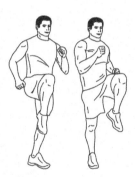

20 high knees

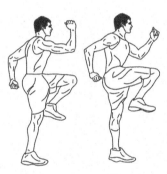

20 march steps

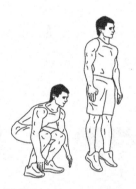

10 jump squats

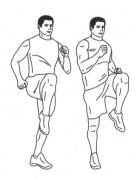

20 high knees

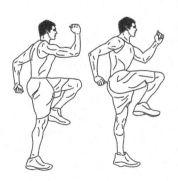

20 march steps

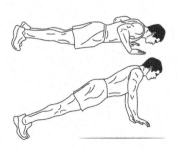

10 power push-ups

11   Body Patch

Body Patch is a full bodyweight high-performance workout that is designed to help you develop strength, core stability and dense, powerful muscles. The exercises are performed in their fullest range of movement with punches utilizing full body movement behind them for extra strength and power.

Focus: Strength & Tone

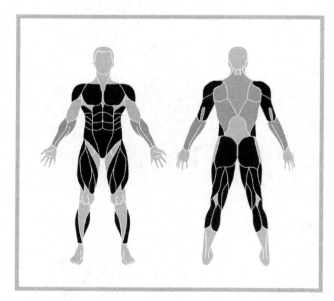

BODY PATCH

DAREBEE WORKOUT
© darebee.com
LEVEL I 3 sets
LEVEL II 5 sets
LEVEL III 7 sets
REST up to 2 minutes

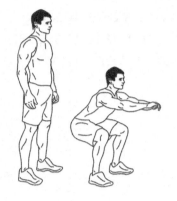

20 squats

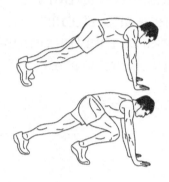

20 slow climbers

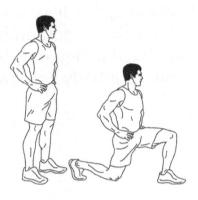

20 lunges

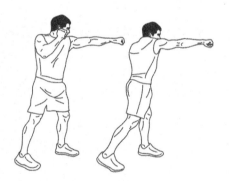

40 punches

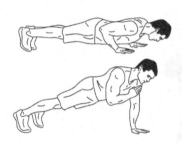

20 push-up shoulder taps

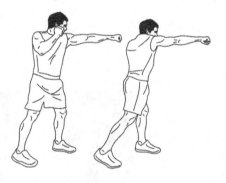

40 punches

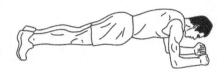

20-count plank

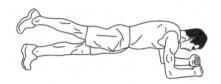

20-count raised leg plank

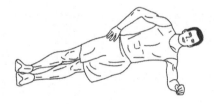

20-count side plank

12 Bootcamp

When you start the Bootcamp workout you realize just why it's called Bootcamp. Each exercise is designed to build on the previous one, testing strength and endurance, balance and stability, coordination and technique. With overlapping muscles working, this becomes the kind of workout you know your body will know it did the day after.

Focus: Strength & Tone

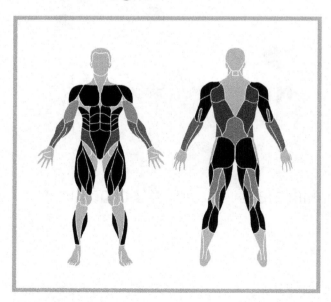

BOOTCAMP

DAREBEE WORKOUT © darebee.com

LEVEL I 3 sets **LEVEL II** 5 sets **LEVEL III** 7 sets **REST** up to 2 minutes

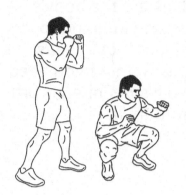
20 squats

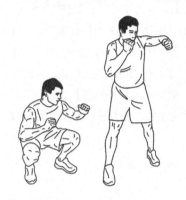
20 squat + hook

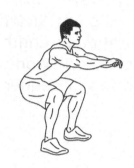
20-count squat hold

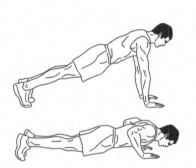
10 push-ups

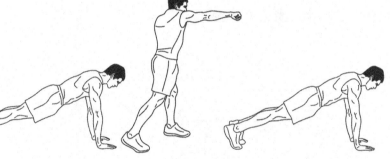
10 plank step-out + punches

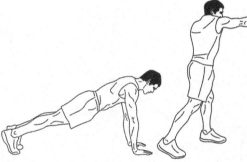
10-count plank

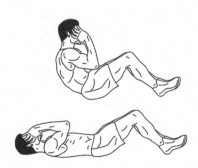
10 sit-ups

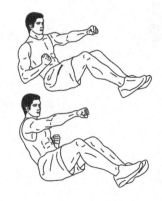
10 sit-up + punches

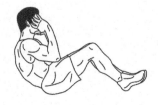
10-count sit-up hold

13 Bottom Line

Glutes, quads, hamstrings, lower body tendons and calves are the body's natural power core. They power everything from running and jumping to punching and kicking. The Bottom Line workout targets just these areas generating strength that will be converted into power the moment you need it. This is one workout you should never really tire of and it's definitely worth returning to frequently and yes ... that EC. Do not forget to try it.

Focus: Strength & Tone

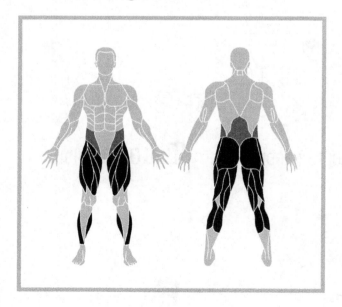

THE BOTTOM LINE

DAREBEE WORKOUT
FOR LEGS & BUTTOCKS
© darebee.com

LEVEL I 3 sets
LEVEL II 4 sets
LEVEL III 5 sets
REST 2 minutes

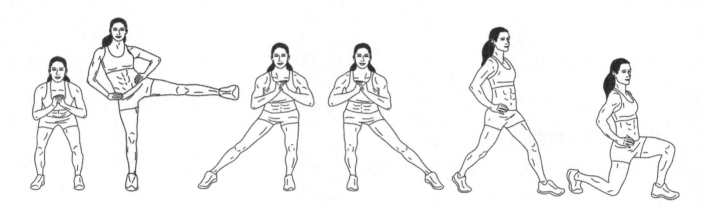

20 squat + side leg raise   **20** side-to-side lunges   **20** split lunges

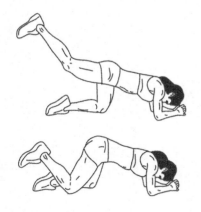 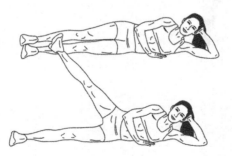 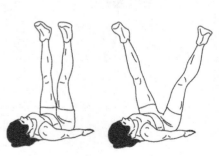

20 plank back kicks   **20** side leg raises   **20** split wipers

14 Bounty Hunter

There is an easy way to make a workout hard: alternate between static and ballistic movements, loading the muscles with bodyweight and then asking them to explode and move through their full range of motion when they are already tired. If that sounds a tad hard it is because, it is. It is also highly effective delivering a high-burn body-shaping workout you really feel working five minutes in.

Focus: Strength & Tone

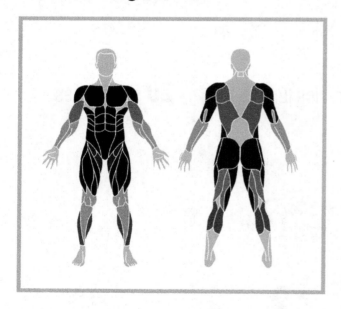

BOUNTY HUNTER

DAREBEE WORKOUT
© darebee.com
LEVEL I 3 sets
LEVEL II 5 sets
LEVEL III 7 sets
REST up to 2 minutes

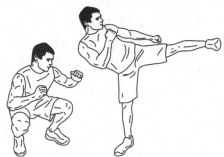

20 squat + side kick

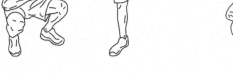

4 side-to-side lunges

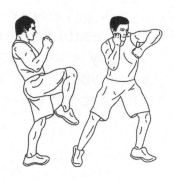

20 knee strike + elbow strike

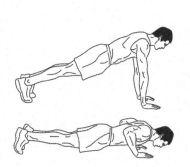

20 push-ups

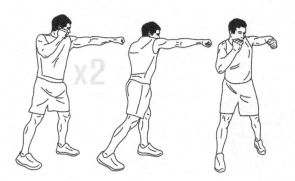

20 jab + jab + cross + hook

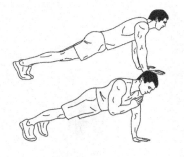

20 shoulder taps

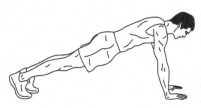

10 up and down planks

+

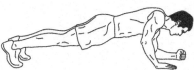 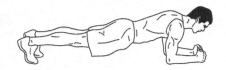

10-count elbow plank hold finish

15   Boxer Abs

Boxing without abs work is like trying to row without a paddle. You will simply not get anywhere fast. Boxer Abs addresses this through nine exercises that target the four muscle groups that make us the abdominals. If you really want to train like a boxer here you will forego the rest and simply let your abs scream for a while. Yo will most definitely see and feel the difference in your overall performance.

Focus: Abs

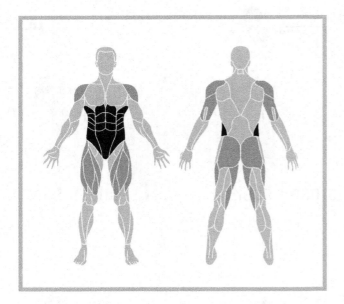

BOXER | ABS

DAREBEE BOXING WORKOUT © darebee.com

LEVEL I 3 sets **LEVEL II** 4 sets **LEVEL III** 5 sets **REST** 2 minutes

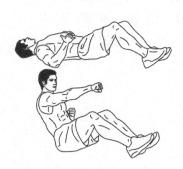

30 sit-up punches

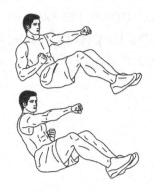

30 siting punches

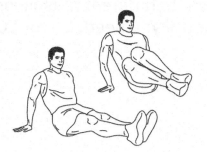

30 knee-ins & twists

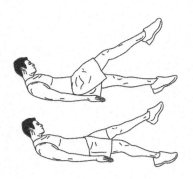

30 flutter kicks

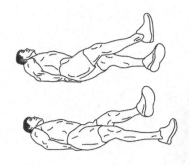

30 scissors

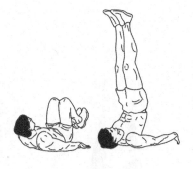

30 butt-ups

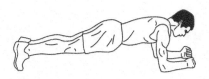

30-count plank

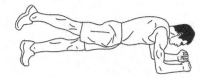

30-count raised leg plank

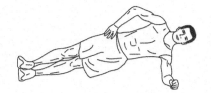

30-count side plank

16 Boxer Flexibility

Boxing requires the body to work with the efficiency of a coiled spring and the fluidity of a panther and that requires flexibility. Not just that of tendons but fascial flexibility as well as loose, relaxed muscles. Boxer Flexibility recruits different muscle groups to provide the kind of suppleness and control you need. Go for EC. Your body will thank you for it later.

Focus: Stretching

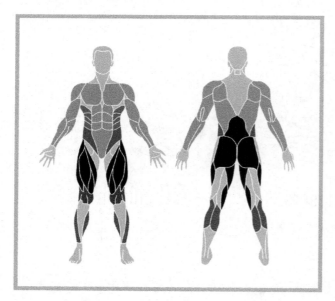

BOXER |
FLEXIBILITY

DAREBEE BOXING WORKOUT © darebee.com
LEVEL I 3 sets **LEVEL II** 4 sets **LEVEL III** 5 sets
REST 2 minutes

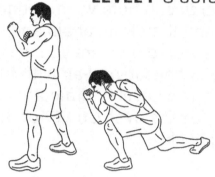

40 knee-to-elbow lunges

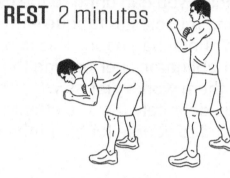

20 forward & backward bends

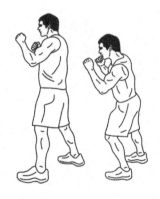

20 side-to-side tilts

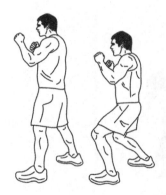

20 knee bends

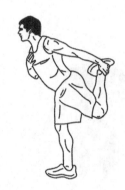

40-count quad stretch

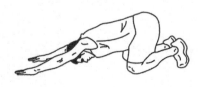

20-count back stretch

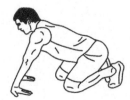

20-count arm stretch #1

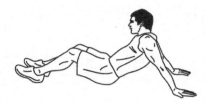

20-count arm stretch #2

17 Boxer Power

Power in boxing is a multi-factorial outcome which is a fancy way of saying that if you want to pack more power than a newborn kitten you'd better be prepared to train your socks off. Every muscle counts so Boxer Power recruits all the muscles you can bring to the exercise. It puts you through your paces by forcing muscles to fatigue early and then train again and again. If you have a punch bag handy this is one workout where you get to use it, but it's not obligatory, performing the punches in mid-air with full body swing behind them works just as well. This is a Level IV difficulty workout and you will definitely feel the effects after it's over. Go EC for the extra burn and be kind to yourself: hold nothing back!

Focus: Strength & Tone

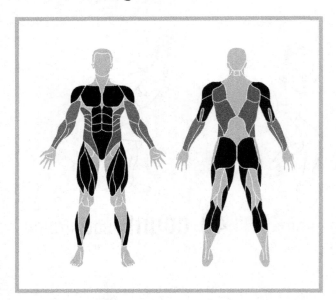

BOXER|POWER

DAREBEE BOXING WORKOUT © darebee.com
LEVEL I 3 sets LEVEL II 4 sets LEVEL III 5 sets REST 2 minutes
tip: last row can be done on a punching bag

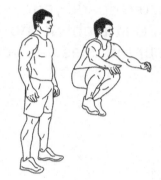 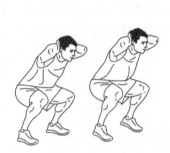 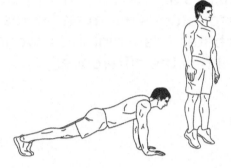

20 jump knee tucks   **20** squat hops   **20** basic burpees + jump

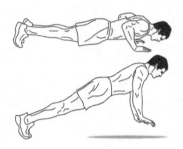 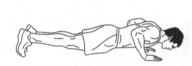 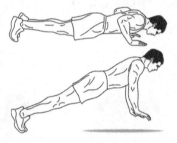

10 power push-ups   **10-count** push-up plank   **10** power push-ups

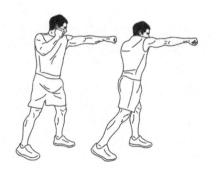 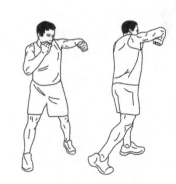 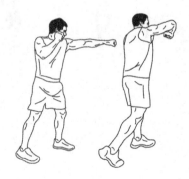

40 jab + cross   **40** hooks (left + right)   **40** jab + hook

18   Cardio Combat

Combat and cardio were made for each other which is why Cardio Combat pushes all the skeletal muscle fast-response buttons, overloads your respiratory system and screams for you to do it with EC straight up, no debates. It's a high burn workout. It will streamline your muscles and you will feel the difference.

Focus: High Burn

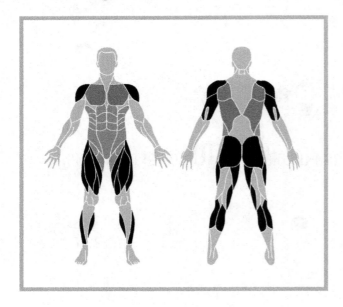

CARDIO COMBAT

DAREBEE WORKOUT
© darebee.com
LEVEL I 3 sets
LEVEL II 5 sets
LEVEL III 7 sets
REST up to 2 minutes

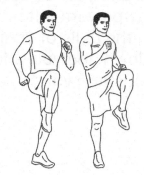

20 high knees

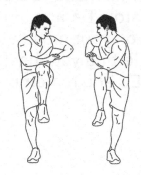

10 march twists

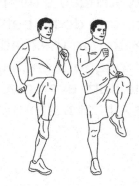

20 high knees

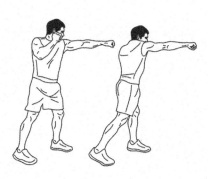

20 punches

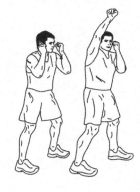

10 overhead punches

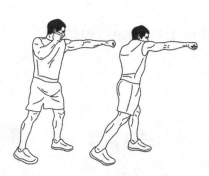

20 punches

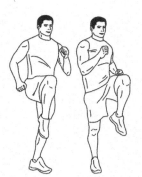

20 high knees

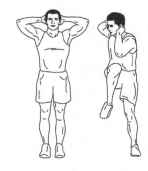

10 knee-to-elbow

one side first, then the other side

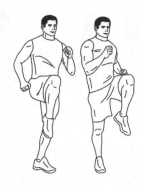

20 high knees

19 Cardio Demon

When you need a high burn that will make your heart race and your sweat run you can do no better than Cardio Demon. It is fast. It is powerful. It is unrelenting in the load it places on your muscles. Stay on the balls of your feet throughout each set, never letting your heels touch down and you will feel the burn even more. Go for EC and remember this is pushing you to new levels of performance.

Focus: High Burn

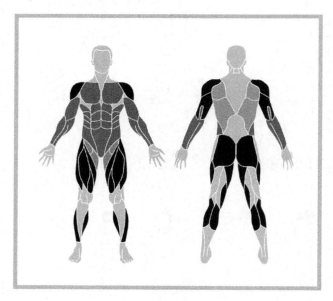

CARDIO DEMON

DAREBEE WORKOUT
© darebee.com
LEVEL I 3 sets
LEVEL II 5 sets
LEVEL III 7 sets
REST up to 2 minutes

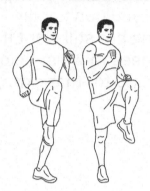

20 high knees

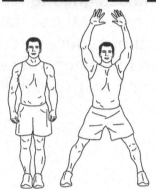

20 jumping jacks

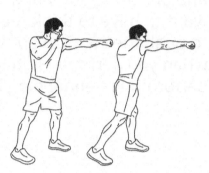

20 punches

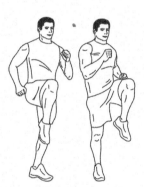

20 high knees

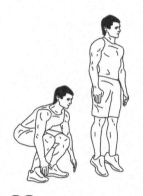

20 jump squats

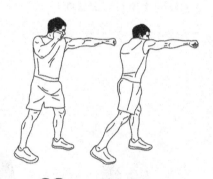

20 punches

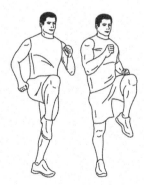

20 high knees

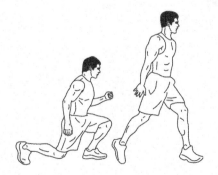

20 jumping lunges

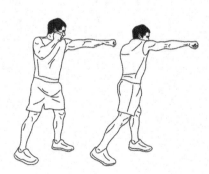

20 punches

20 Cardio Drill

Cardio Drill is fast, energetic and designed to test your VO2 Max capacity and open up your lungs. It's perfect for those days when you don't really want to have to think too hard about your exercise routine but still want it to push the envelope of your performance. Raise your knees to waist height when you perform High Knees and try to get it done with EC for that extra, performance-enhancing burn.

Focus: High Burn

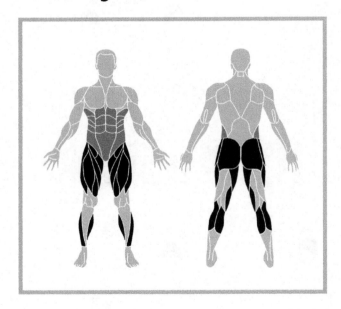

CARDIO DRILL

DAREBEE WORKOUT © darebee.com

Level I 3 sets **Level II** 5 sets **Level III** 7 sets **REST** up to 2 minutes

3combos:

20 high knees
4 knee-to-elbow

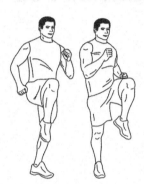
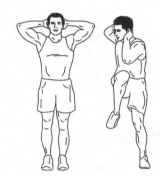

3combos:

20 high knees
2 side-to-side jumps

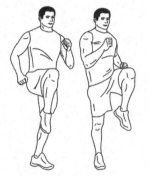
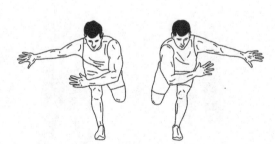

3combos:

20 high knees
4 side leg raises

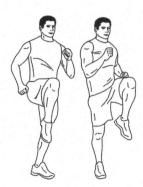
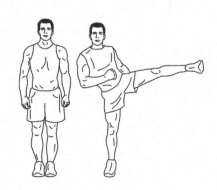

21 Cardio Fire

Because we are grounded by gravity and can neither fly nor levitate our legs power everything. We use them to jump, run, walk, stand and fight. The power of punches and how hard we can push, twist and swing requires good leg strength. The Cardio Fire workout works your lower body, recruiting secondary as well as primary muscle groups and tendons to give you more power in your future physical activities.

Focus: High Burn

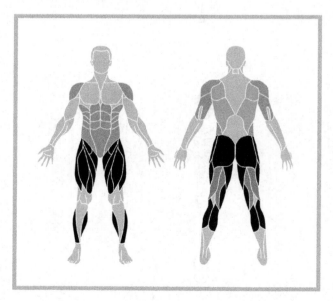

CARDIO FIRE

WORKOUT
BY DAREBEE
© darebee.com

LEVEL I 3 sets
LEVEL II 5 sets
LEVEL III 7 sets
2 minutes rest

10 jumping jacks

4 side-to-side jumps

10 jumping jacks

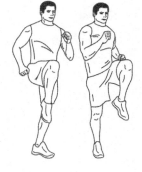

10 high knees

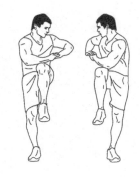

4 knee-to-elbow twists

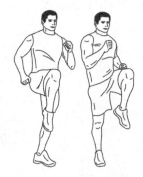

10 high knees

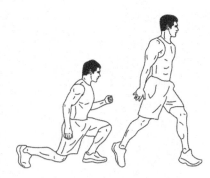

10 jumping lunges

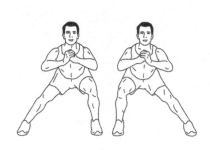

4 side-to-side lunges

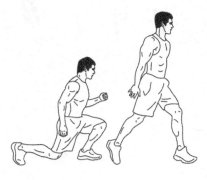

10 jumping lunges

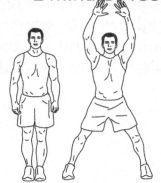

22   Cardio Light

There are times when you want to workout and barely have the energy to get going. For those times the Cardio Light, will get you buzzing in just the right way. Designed to get your body going and your heart thumping without pushing you too hard, this is just the kind of go-to workout you go to, when you're low and really need a pick-me-up.

Focus: High Burn

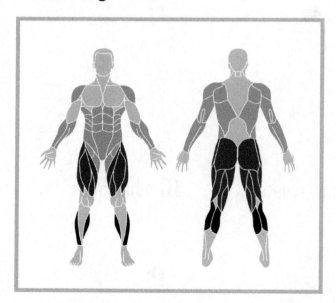

cardio light

DAREBEE WORKOUT © darebee.com

LEVEL I 3 sets **LEVEL II** 5 sets **LEVEL III** 7 sets **REST** up to 2 minutes

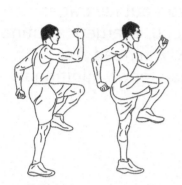

10 march steps

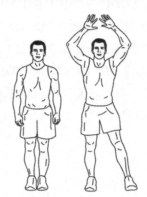

20 step jacks

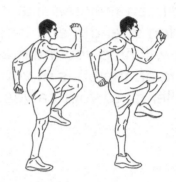

10 march steps

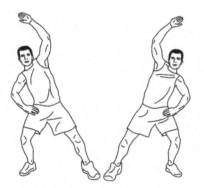

20 side jacks

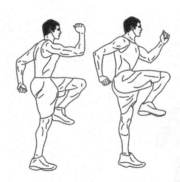

10 march steps

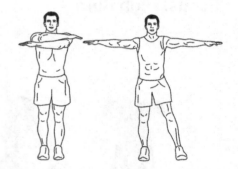

20 scissor steps

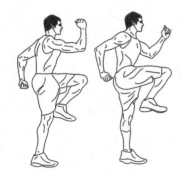

10 march steps

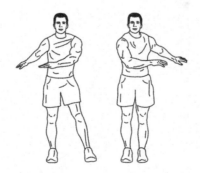

20 side-to-side steps

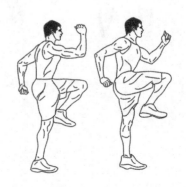

10 march steps

23 Cardio Melt

Cardio Melt will not necessarily melt your heart but do it fast enough and it will certainly feel like it's what it's trying to do. The workout leverages tendon strength and fascial fitness to create a fast-paced, energetic routine that will help you maintain the physical edge you know you need. Try being on the balls of your feet throughout every exercise for an additional challenge to your calves and core.

Focus: High Burn

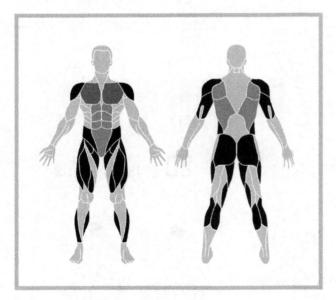

cardio melt

DAREBEE WORKOUT © darebee.com

Level I 3 sets **Level II** 5 sets **Level III** 7 sets **REST** 2 minutes rest

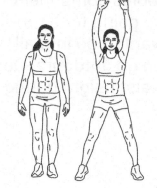

20 jumping jacks

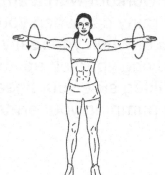

20 arm circles

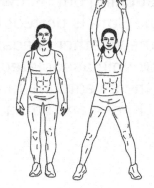

20 jumping jacks

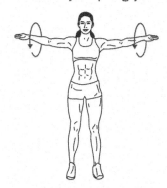

20 arm circles

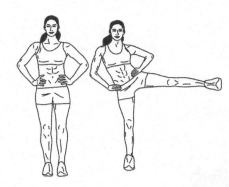

20 side leg raises

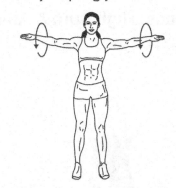

20 arm circles

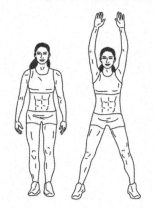

20 jumping jacks

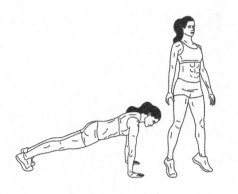

20 basic burpees

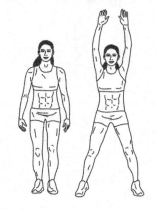

20 jumping jacks

24 Cardio Sofa

The Cardio Sofa workout uses your sofa for something decidedly different to couching out. A lower body workout with a strong aerobics component Cardio Sofa is perfect for that rainy day when you feel like going for a run but the weather is against you or when you really don't want to go into all the trouble associated with tidying yourself up so you can go outdoors. Get into the sweatzone fast by making sure your knees are waist height during High Knees and you are really pumping your arms.

Focus: High Burn & Abs

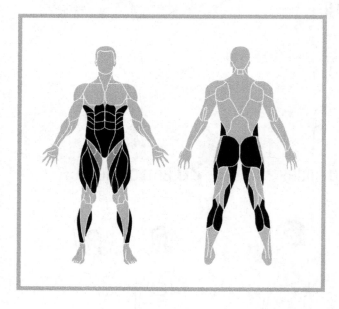

cardio sofa

DAREBEE WORKOUT © darebee.com

LEVEL I 3 sets **LEVEL II** 5 sets **LEVEL III** 7 sets **REST** 2 minutes

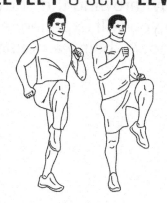

40 high knees

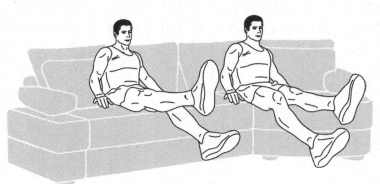

20 flutter kicks

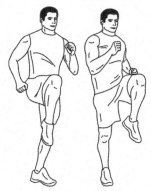

40 high knees

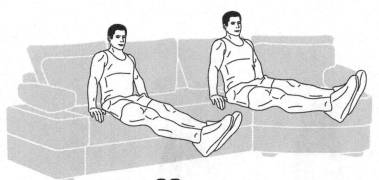

20 leg raises

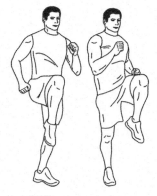

40 high knees

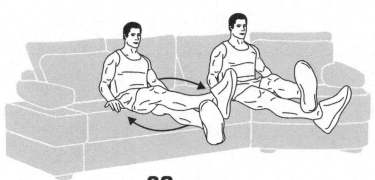

20 scissors

25 Caterpillar-Butterfly

If it's fascial fitness you want and powerful tendons, then the Caterpillar-Butterfly workout will be a transforming experience. By throwing the body about like it has no mass and gravity has no meaning you will experience the exhilaration of total control and the sensation of power being amplified.

Focus: High Burn

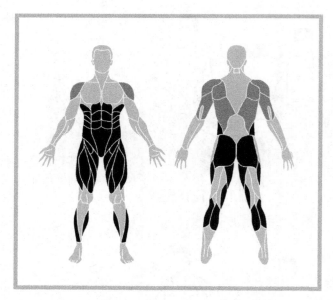

caterpillar-
Butterfly

DAREBEE WORKOUT © **darebee.com**

LEVEL I 3 sets **LEVEL II** 5 sets **LEVEL III** 7 sets **REST** up to 2 minutes

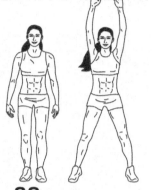

20 jumping jacks

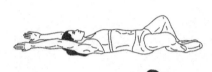

10 butterfly sit-ups

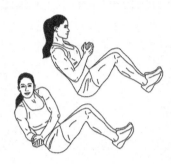

10 sitting twists

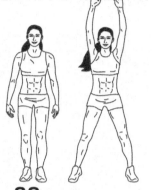

20 jumping jacks

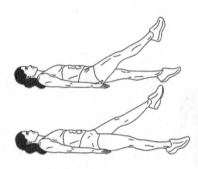

10 flutter kicks

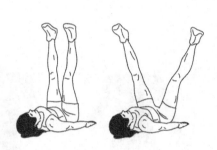

10 V-wipers

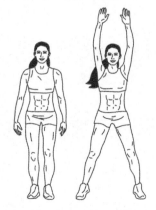

20 jumping jacks

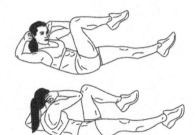

10 knee-to-elbow crunches

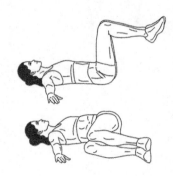

10 half wipers

26 Centurion

In the ancient world fitness was a necessity rather than a pastime. The Centurion workout aims at functional fitness targeting the muscles used by the body when it needs to move fast, jump far and fight.

Focus: Strength & Tone

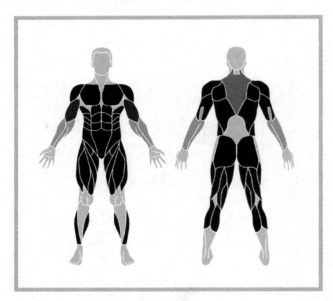

CENTURION

DAREBEE WORKOUT © darebee.com

LEVEL I 3 sets **LEVEL II** 5 sets **LEVEL III** 7 sets **REST** up to 2 minutes

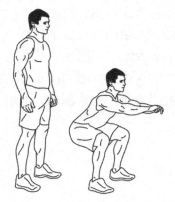
10combo squat + calf raise

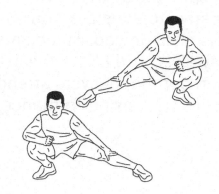
10 side-to-side lunges

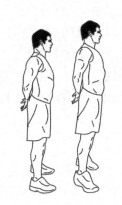
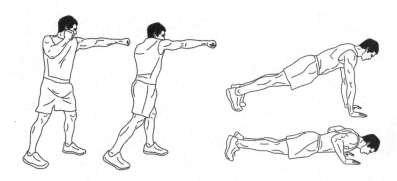
10combo jab + cross + push-up

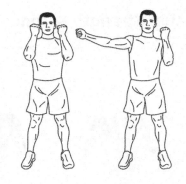
10 side-to-side backfists

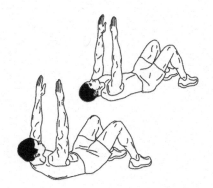
10 high crunches

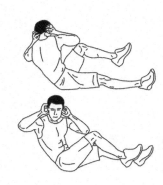
10 knee-to-elbow crunches

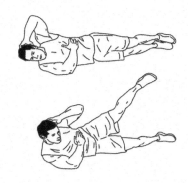
10 side jackknives

27 Cerberus

Despite the dexterity with which we can use it our upper body strength, relative to the size of our body, is pretty weak. Cerberus tries to address this all in one go, which should be a hint for you on how you will feel the day after. Add EC for the extra bite (pun unintended) and you end up with a workout that delivers strength, can help with limb speed and will also test your VO2 Max performance, too.

Focus: Strength & Tone

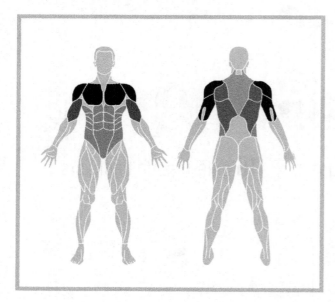

CERBERUS

DAREBEE WORKOUT © darebee.com

LEVEL I 3 sets **LEVEL II** 5 sets **LEVEL III** 7 sets **REST** up to 2 minutes

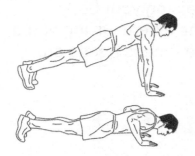

6 push-ups

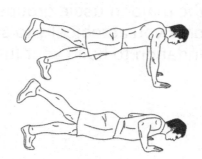

4 raised leg push-ups

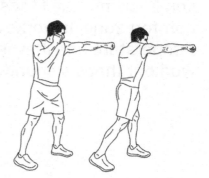

20 punches

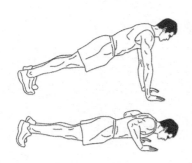

6 push-ups

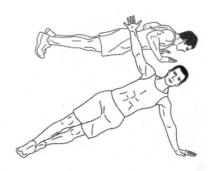

4 push-ups w/ rotations

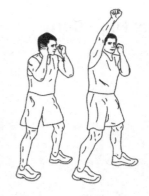

20 overhead punches

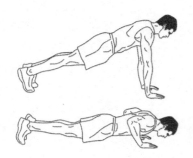

6 push-ups

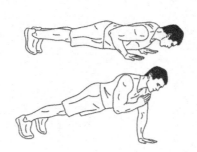

4 shoulder taps

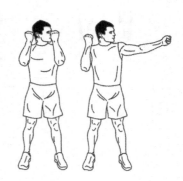

20 backfists

Chapter 1

Everyone deserves a fresh start and the Chapter 1 workout gently eases you back into the fitness groove without forcing you too far from your comfort zone. It works all the major muscle groups, raising your body temperature and it even works you aerobically to some extent, giving you a workout that's a sound foundation to build your future fitness needs on.

Focus: High Burn

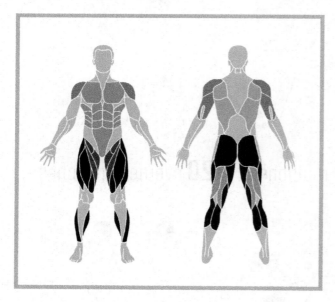

Chapter 1

DAREBEE WORKOUT © darebee.com

LEVEL I 3 sets **LEVEL II** 5 sets **LEVEL III** 7 sets **REST** up to 2 minutes

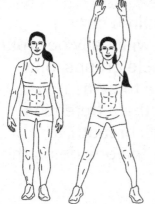

20 jumping jacks

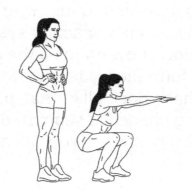

10 squats

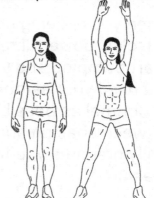

20 jumping jacks

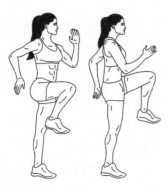

10 march steps

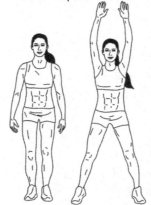

20 jumping jacks

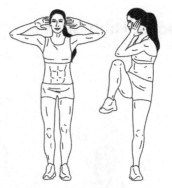

10 knee-to-elbow

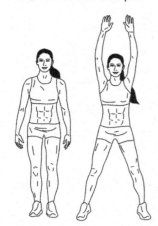

20 jumping jacks

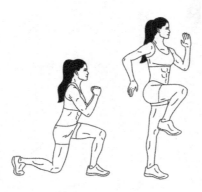

10 lunge step-up

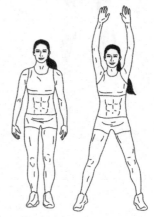

20 jumping jacks

29 Chase

When you're being chased you need to run. Your body requires strong muscles, powerful tendons, a cardiovascular system that will really get your heart pumping and your blood flowing to all the right muscle groups, plus you need your aerobic performance, your VO2 Max volume to be as near as optimal as possible. Chase does all of that, plus, since the difference between chasing and being chased is separated by a hair's breadth, it really prepares you for the times when you will need to be the one doing the chasing.

Focus: High Burn

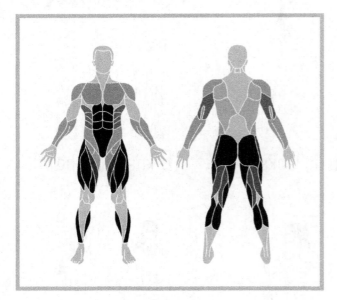

CHASE

DAREBEE WORKOUT © darebee.com

LEVEL I 3 sets **LEVEL II** 5 sets **LEVEL III** 7 sets **REST** up to 2 minutes

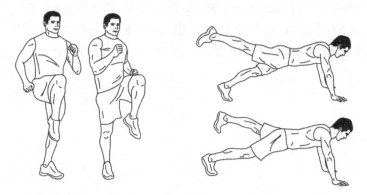

3combos: **10** high knees + **4** plank leg raises

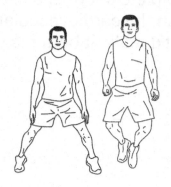

10 hop heel clicks

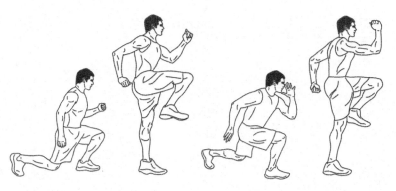

10combos successive lunge step-ups

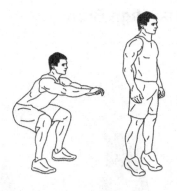

10 squat calf raises

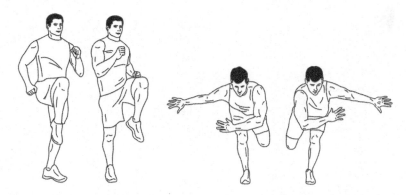

3combos: **10** high knees + **4** side-to-side hops

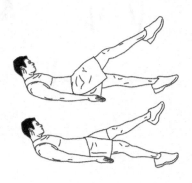

40 flutter kicks

30 Chimera

The Chimera workout is a mixed beast of a fitness routine. It uses a complete set of exercise to challenge tendon strength, activate muscles, push the cardiovascular system and make the core stronger. The only thing that'd make it better is your doing the entire routine at level III, twice.

Focus: High Burn

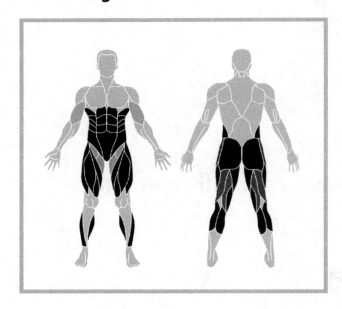

CHIMERA

DAREBEE WORKOUT © darebee.com

LEVEL I 3 sets **LEVEL II** 5 sets **LEVEL III** 7 sets **REST** up to 2 minutes

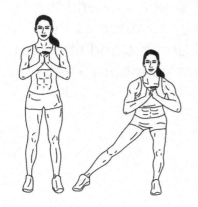

20 side-to-side lunges

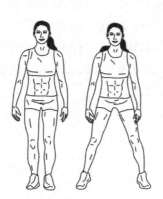

20combos half jack + side leg raise

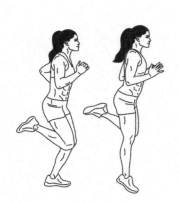

10 butt kicks

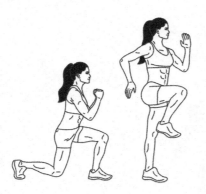

10 lunge step-ups

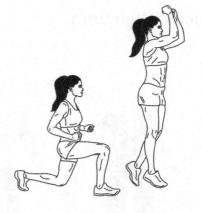

10 jumping lunges

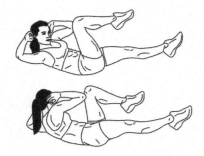

10 knee-to-elbow crunches

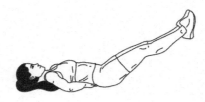

10-count raised leg hold

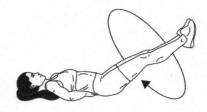

10 raised leg circles

31 Chisel

Getting that chiseled physique requires patience, perseverance and the ability to put in the time one day after another. Chisel, of course, is the workout that'll help you do all this. A combination of aerobic and strength exercises it works all the major muscle groups so that your body keeps on changing the way you want it to.

Focus: High Burn

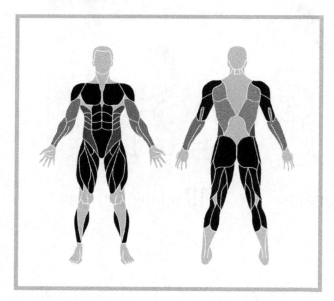

CHISEL

DAREBEE WORKOUT © darebee.com

LEVEL I 3 sets **LEVEL II** 5 sets **LEVEL III** 7 sets **REST** up to 2 minutes

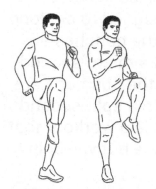

20 high knees

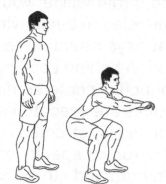

10 squats

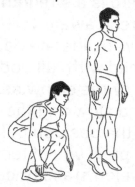

10 jump squats

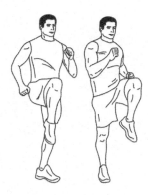

20 high knees

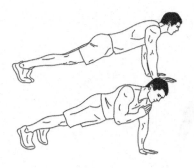

10 shoulder taps

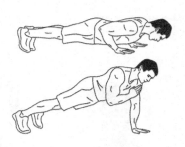

10 shoulder tap push-ups

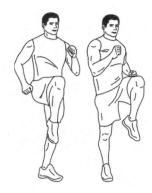

20 high knees

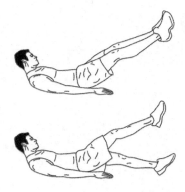

10 flutter kicks

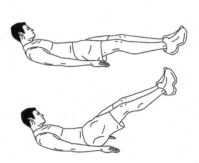

10 leg raises

32   Code Zero

Code Zero is a strength workout that will let you feel muscles in places you weren't aware you had muscles to begin with. It's designed to be done at a slow, deliberate pace that pays attention to form so the punches are performed with full body rotation behind each punch and a micro-second locking of the elbow as the punch is centered each time, the push ups are deep and slow and the side kicks are executed slowly with a split-second hold of the position before the leg is retracted. The result is a workout that will not push you in terms of aerobic capacity or endurance but will help you develop stability, core strength and strong muscles.

Focus: Strength & Tone

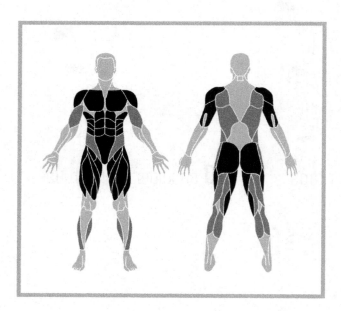

CODE ZERO

DAREBEE WORKOUT © darebee.com

LEVEL I 3 sets **LEVEL II** 5 sets **LEVEL III** 7 sets **REST** up to 2 minutes

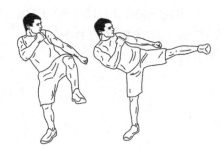

20 side kicks

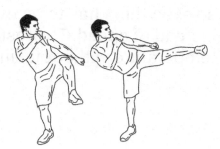

5 push-ups

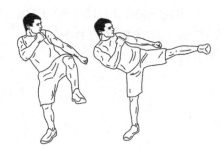

20 side kicks

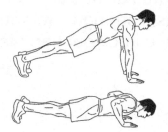

20 punches

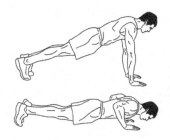

5 push-ups

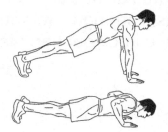

20 punches

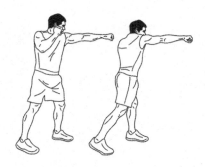

20-count elbow plank

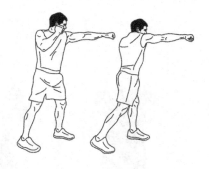

5 push-ups

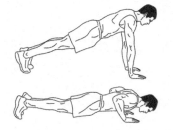

20-count elbow plank

33 Commander

The Commander is a strength training workout that uses the dynamic movement of punches in combination with exercises to test almost every muscle group in the body. The emphasis here is on full body movement so everything has to be executed using correct form and deep movement, instead of speed. The result is a strength workout that raises the body temperature without taking you into your aerobic zone.

Focus: Strength & Tone

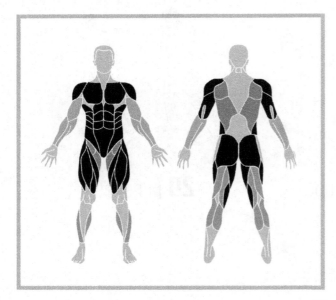

THE COMMANDER

DAREBEE WORKOUT © darebee.com

LEVEL I 3 sets **LEVEL II** 5 sets **LEVEL III** 7 sets **REST** up to 2 minutes

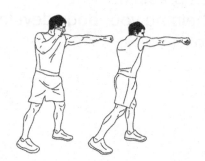

40 jab + cross

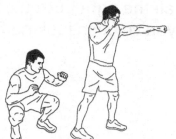

20 squat + jab

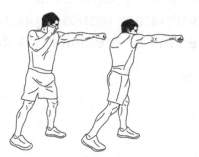

40 jab + cross

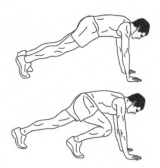

20 slow climber

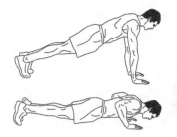

20 push-ups

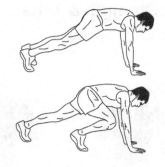

20 slow climbers

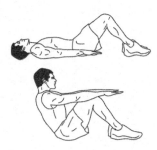

20 sit-ups

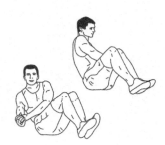

20 sitting twists

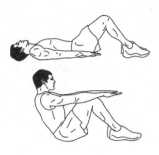

20 sit-ups

34 Commando

There are times when what you want is your body to obey you, explicitly. You want your muscles to respond quickly and with precision. The Commando workout pushes all the right buttons, helping your body develop the kind of precision control you've been looking for.

Focus: Strength & Tone

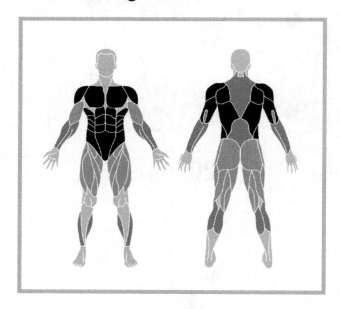

COMMANDO

DAREBEE WORKOUT © darebee.com

LEVEL I 3 sets **LEVEL II** 4 sets **LEVEL III** 5 sets **REST** up to 2 minutes

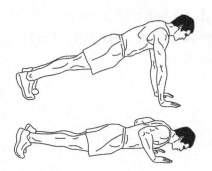

to failure push-ups

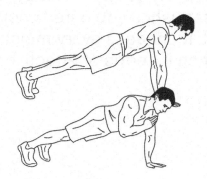

10 shoulder taps

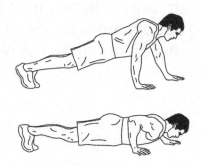

4 staggered push-ups

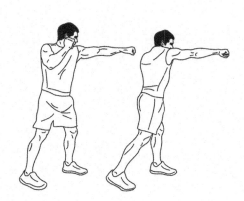

40 punches

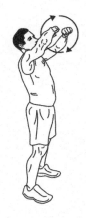

40 speed bag punches

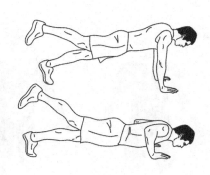

4 raised leg push-ups

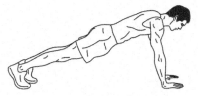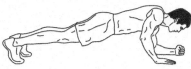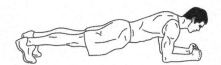

10 up and down planks

35 Conqueror

Conqueror is the workout you go to when you don't really feel like working out. It looks and feels deceptively easy. Its steady rate of work builds up steam gradually but it never pushes you hared enough to feel you have to dig deep to complete it. Yet, it engages every major muscle group you have and it delivers quite the punch in terms of effectiveness.

Focus: Strength & Tone

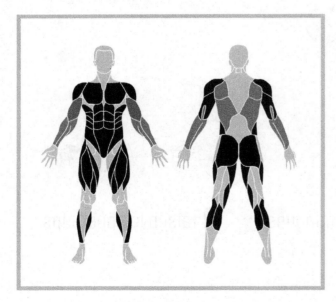

CONQUEROR

DAREBEE WORKOUT © darebee.com

LEVEL I 3 sets **LEVEL II** 5 sets **LEVEL III** 7 sets **REST** up to 2 minutes

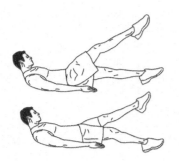

20 squats

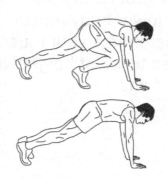

20 slow climbers

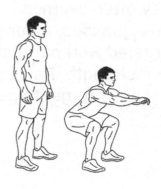

20 squats

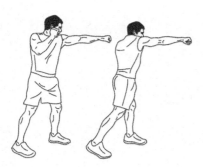

20 punches

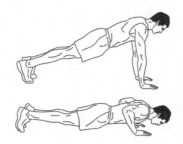

20 push-ups

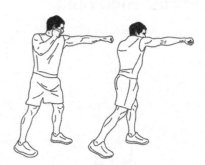

20 punches

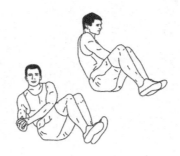

20 flutter kicks

20 sitting twists

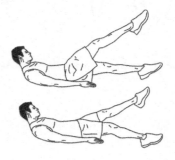

20 flutter kicks

36 Cossack

Cossacks were light on their feet and had such famously strong legs that they often seemed to fly above ground in battle. Cossack, as you might have guessed, focuses on the lower body muscles to deliver a powerful, targeted workout that will supercharge your muscles and help increase your strength. Raise your knees to waist height when doing March Steps and don't forget to pump your arms.

Focus: High Burn

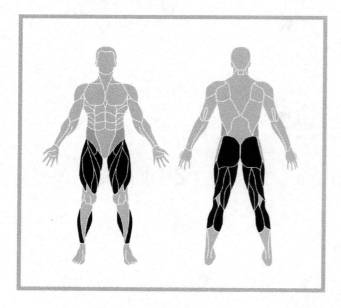

cossack

DAREBEE WORKOUT © darebee.com

Level I 3 sets **Level II** 5 sets **Level III** 7 sets **REST** 2 minutes

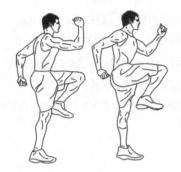

20 march steps

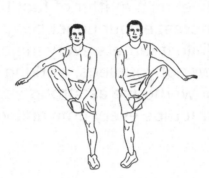

10 toe tap hops

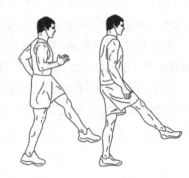

20 straight leg bounds

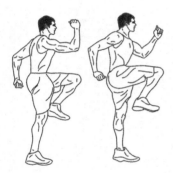

20 march steps

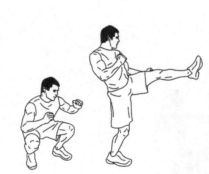

10 squat + front kick

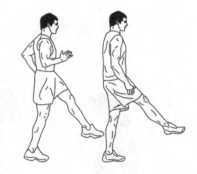

20 straight leg bounds

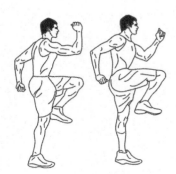

20 march steps

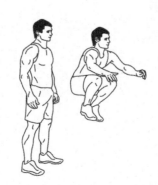

10 jump knee-tucks

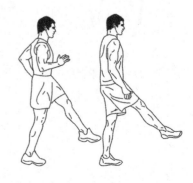

20 straight leg bounds

37 Crusher

Here's a truism: without lower body strength you can do very little. You cannot jump. You cannot run. You cannot kick. You cannot punch. You lose so much of your body's power as a matter of fact that the question has to be what can you do to increase your upper body strength? The answer is The Crusher workout. While it targets every major muscle group in your body, it focuses on the power of your legs, working quads, glutes and calves to make your lower body powerhouse as strong as it can possibly be. Maintain the height of your jumps every time and you will feel the burn from the first set.

Focus: Strength & Tone

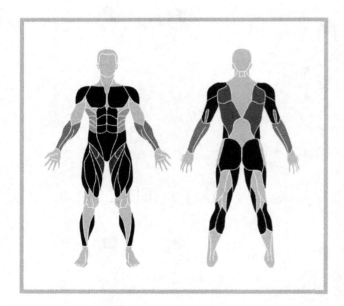

THE CRUSHER

DAREBEE WORKOUT © darebee.com

LEVEL I 3 sets **LEVEL II** 5 sets **LEVEL III** 7 sets **REST** up to 2 minutes

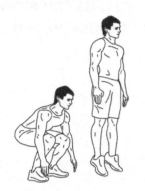

10 jump squats

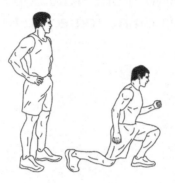

10 lunges

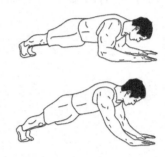

5 tricep extensions

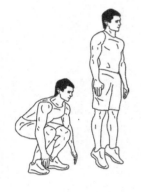

10 jump squats

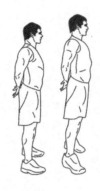

10 calf raises

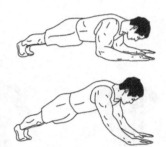

5 tricep extensions

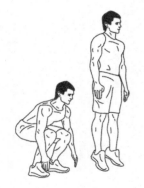

10 jump squats

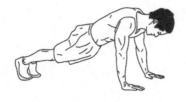

30-count plank

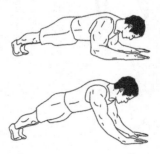

5 tricep extensions

38 Cypher

Decipher your body, up your speed and push your aerobic performance to new heights with the Cypher workout. This combines it all plus the slow exercises at the end of each combo force you to use your muscles fully.

Focus: Strength & Tone

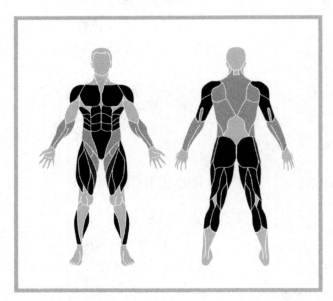

CYPHER

LEVEL I 3 sets **LEVEL II** 5 sets **LEVEL III** 7 sets **REST** up to 2 minutes

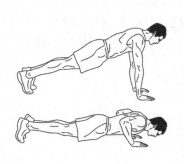 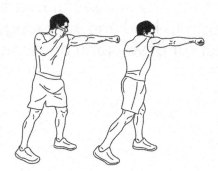 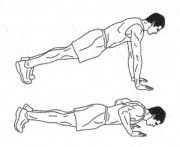

4combos: **2** push-up + **10** jab + cross   **10** slow push-ups

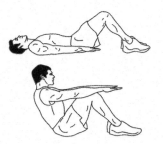 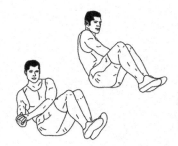 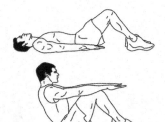

4combos: **2** sit-ups + **10** sitting twists   **10** slow sit-ups

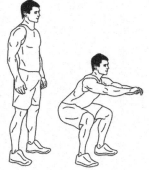 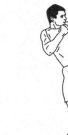 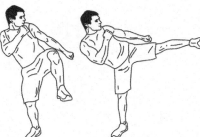 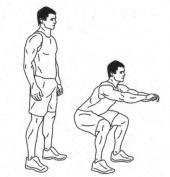

4combos: **2** squats + **10** side kicks   **10** slow squats

39   Damage Control

You can do anything for 10 seconds, right? This is why the Damage Control workout is so awesome. It takes 10 second bursts and piles them on so that your muscles soon begin to load and your lungs to labor. Its fast, furious pace make it perfect for developing better aerobic capacity and fast-twitch action muscle fiber.

Focus: High Burn, HIIT

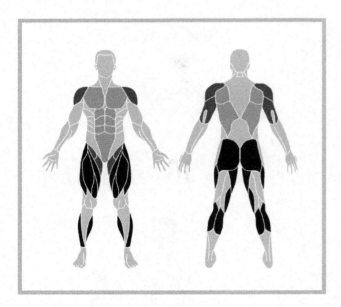

DAMAGE CONTROL

DAREBEE HIIT WORKOUT © darebee.com

Level I 3 sets **Level II** 5 sets **Level III** 7 sets **REST** up to 2 minutes

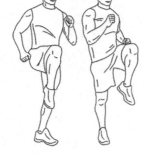
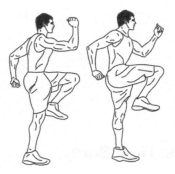

3combos:

10sec high knees
10sec march steps

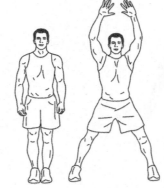
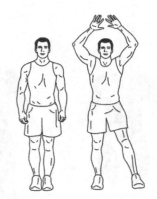

3combos:

10sec jumping jacks
10sec step jacks

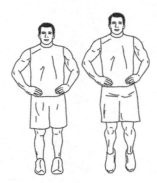
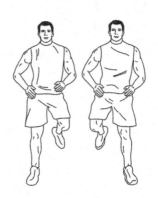

3combos:

10sec hops on the spot
10sec side-to-side hops

40 Danger Zone

Turn your body into an instrument you control at will with the Danger Zone workout. This is both a ballistic and core strength workout focusing on increasing performance because, you know, you really may need those skills when in a tight spot, you know...Danger Zone.

Focus: High Burn

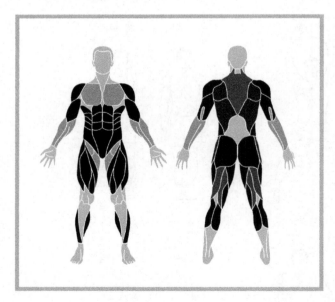

DANGER ZONE

DAREBEE WORKOUT
© darebee.com
LEVEL I 3 sets
LEVEL II 5 sets
LEVEL III 7 sets
REST up to 2 minutes

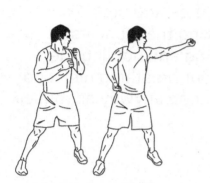 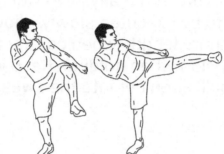 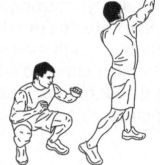

20combos backfist + side kick   **20** squat + uppercut

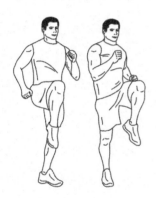 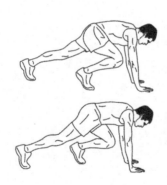 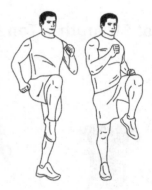

10 high knees   **10** climbers   **10** high knees

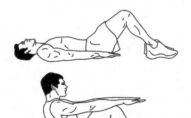 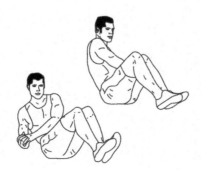 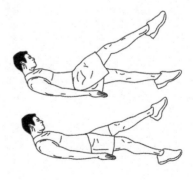

10 sit-ups   **10** sitting twists   **10** flutter kicks

41 Deadlock

Deadlock is an isometric and isotonic workout that helps create better joint stability, a stronger core and really powerful glutes and hips. The exercises are designed to be executed slowly, allowing the muscles to contract through their entire length, when contracting and holding the position in isometric tension when holding. Keep your breathing nice and even throughout and you'll soon get into the sweatzone anyway as muscle temperature rises.

Focus: Strength & Tone

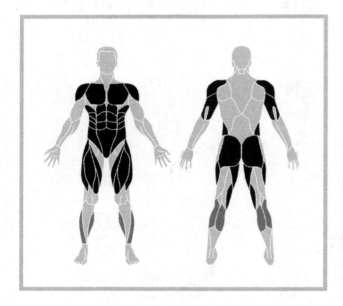

DEADLOCK

DAREBEE WORKOUT © darebee.com

LEVEL I 3 sets **LEVEL II** 5 sets **LEVEL III** 7 sets **REST** up to 2 minutes

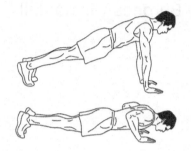

5 push-ups

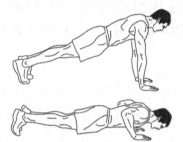

10-count push-up hold

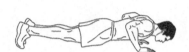

5 push-ups

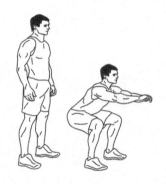

20 squats

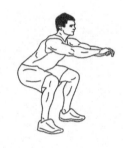

20-count squat hold

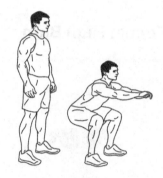

20 squats

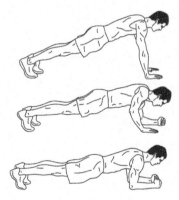

5 up & down planks

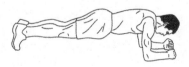

10-count elbow plank hold

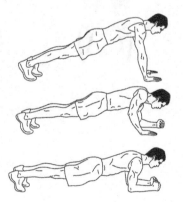

5 up & down planks

42   Death by Burpees

Burpees are your body's fight against gravity. The more you fight, the stronger you get. The stronger you get the more you do. The more you do the higher you fly. The..., you get the picture. Death by Burpees will not kill you. So, it will make you stronger.

Focus: High Burn

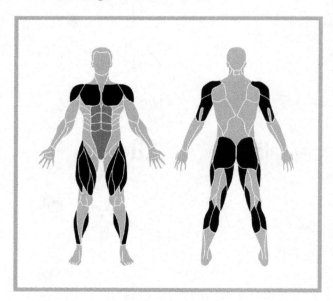

DEATH BY BURPEES

DAREBEE WORKOUT © **darebee.com**
LEVEL I 3 sets **LEVEL II** 4 sets **LEVEL III** 5 sets
2 minutes rest between sets

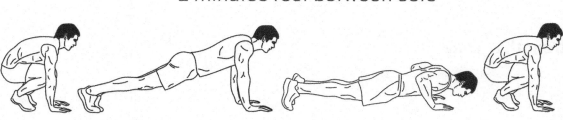

5 burpees	10-count rest
5 burpees	10-count rest
10 burpees	20-count rest
10 burpees	20-count rest
5 burpees	10-count rest
5 burpees	rest

Hint: 10-count rest means count to ten and resume

43   Demolition

Demolition is a level four strength workout that targets the upper body and core and helps you get pumped in no time at all. Do each exercise slowly (including the punches), pay attention to form and go through the full range of motion (which means the push ups are really deep) and you will feel the benefits from all this long before the workout itself is over.

Focus: Strength & Tone

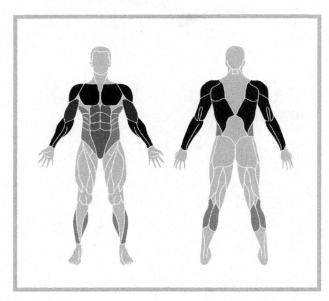

DEMOLITION

DAREBEE WORKOUT © darebee.com

LEVEL I 3 sets **LEVEL II** 4 sets **LEVEL III** 5 sets **REST** up to 2 minutes

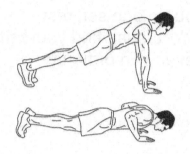

5 classic push-ups

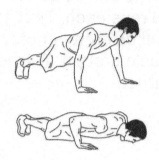

5 wide grip push-ups

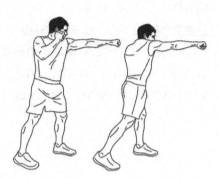

40 punches

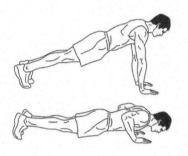

5 classic push-ups

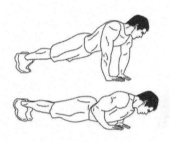

5 close grip push-ups

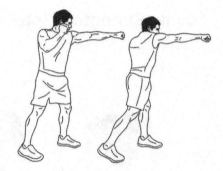

40 punches

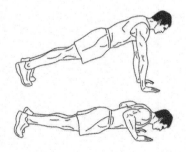

5 classic push-ups

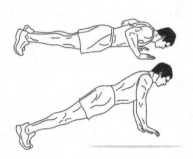

5 power push-ups

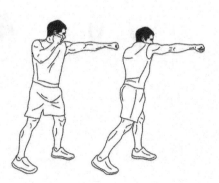

40 punches

44 Dirty 30

For those looking for a quick-and-dirty workout that delivers a punch without too many flourishes none can be quicker or dirtier than Dirty 30. Basically six exercises with 30 reps each. That's it. You do one set, rest, repeat. The results however will be pretty impressive. You shall find yourself working a lot of the major muscle groups. This is a Level IV in difficulty workout, so you have been warned.

Focus: Strength & Tone

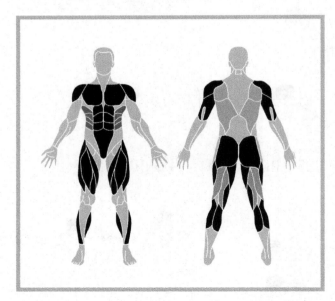

DIRTY 30

DAREBEE WORKOUT © darebee.com

LEVEL I 3 sets **LEVEL II** 4 sets **LEVEL III** 5 sets **REST** up to 2 minutes

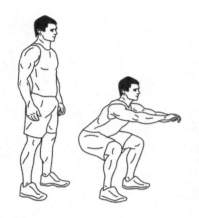

30 squats

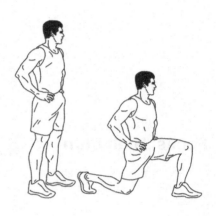

30 push-ups

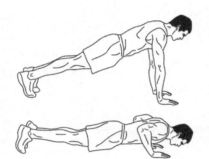

30 lunges

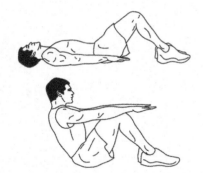

30 sit-ups

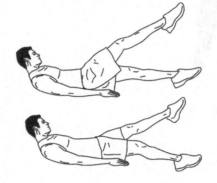

30 flutter kicks

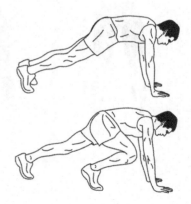

30 climbers

45 Double Dash

Double Dash is a strength workout that alternates the load to the muscles between concentric and eccentric movements, mid-level impact and high impact. As a result it challenges fascial fitness and helps develop the kind of explosive power that transforms your physical performance.

Focus: High Burn

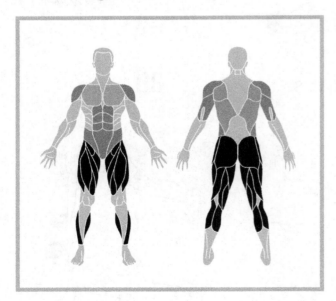

double dash

DAREBEE WORKOUT
© darebee.com
LEVEL I 3 sets
LEVEL II 5 sets
LEVEL III 7 sets
REST up to 2 minutes

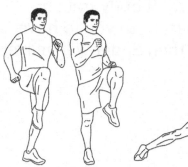
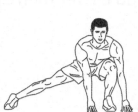

40 high knees   deep side lunge

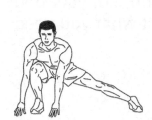
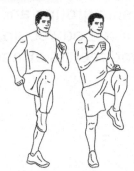

40 high knees   deep side lunge

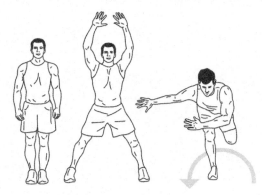

20 jumping jacks   jump to the side

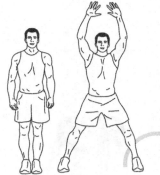
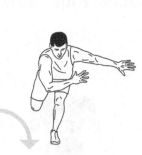

20 jumping jacks   jump to the side

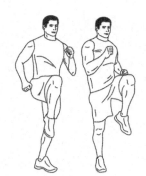
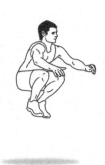

40 high knees   jump knee tuck

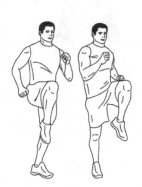
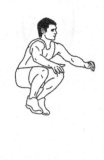

40 high knees   jump knee tuck

46 Ender

Ender is a full body workout that uses a series of standard exercises to challenge specific muscle groups and deliver a near total-body training experience. If you are into body sculpting. If it's important to you to have control of your body and feel its strength and power then Ender will deliver just what you need.

Focus: High Burn

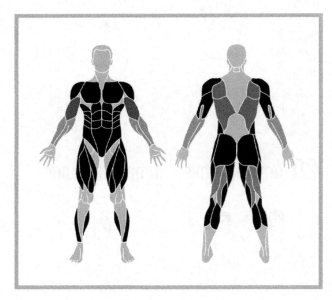

ENDER

DAREBEE WORKOUT © darebee.com

LEVEL I 3 sets **LEVEL II** 5 sets **LEVEL III** 7 sets **REST** up to 2 minutes

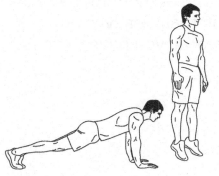

10 basic burpees w/ jump

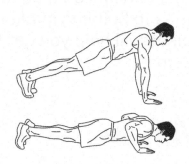

5 push-ups

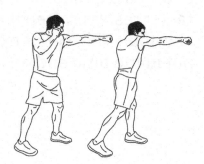

20 punches

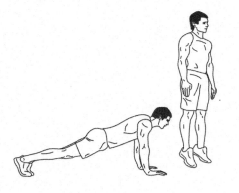

10 basic burpees w/ jump

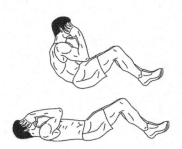

5 sit-ups

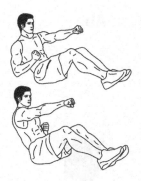

20 sitting punches

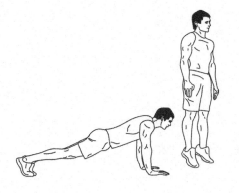

10 basic burpees w/ jump

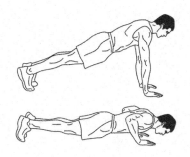

5 push-ups

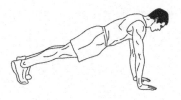

20sec plank

47   Express Abs

There are four main muscle groups that make up the ab wall in its totality and Abs Express is designed to help you test each one of them for better, faster results. When it comes to building quality abs there really is no shortcut. This set of exercises will help you get there, all you have to do is put in the time and do the work.

Focus: Abs

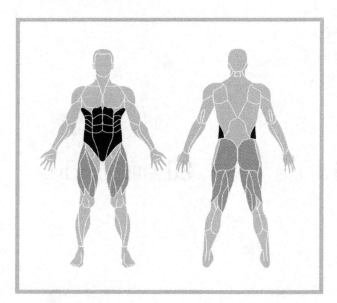

express abs

REPEAT ONCE | DAREBEE WORKOUT © darebee.com
LEVEL I 6 reps **LEVEL II** 10 reps each **LEVEL III** 20 reps each
LEVEL I 6-count hold **LEVEL II** 10-count hold **LEVEL III** 20-count hold

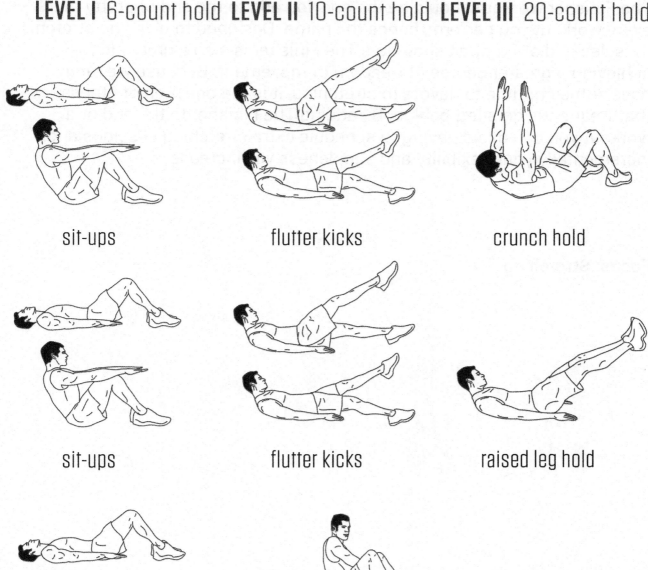

sit-ups   flutter kicks   crunch hold

sit-ups   flutter kicks   raised leg hold

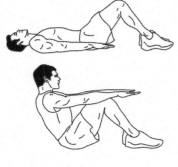

sit-ups   sitting twists   hollow hold

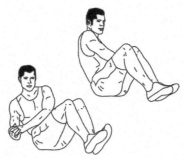

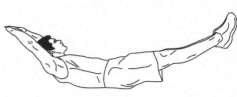

48   Finisher

The Finisher workout should be the one you add to the end of pretty much every workout you perform, hence the name. Designed to help you stretch muscles and strengthen shoulders The Finisher is also a great aid to achieving a greater degree of freedom of movement. Because we rarely have sufficient time to devote to stretching, it is the one area of fitness that frequently gets left behind. By adding The Finisher to the end of a workout you can avoid having to schedule extra stretching sessions and, incrementally your flexibility and suppleness will increase.

Focus: Stretching

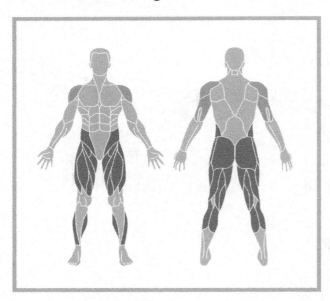

THE FINISHER

STRETCHING BY DAREBEE © darebee.com

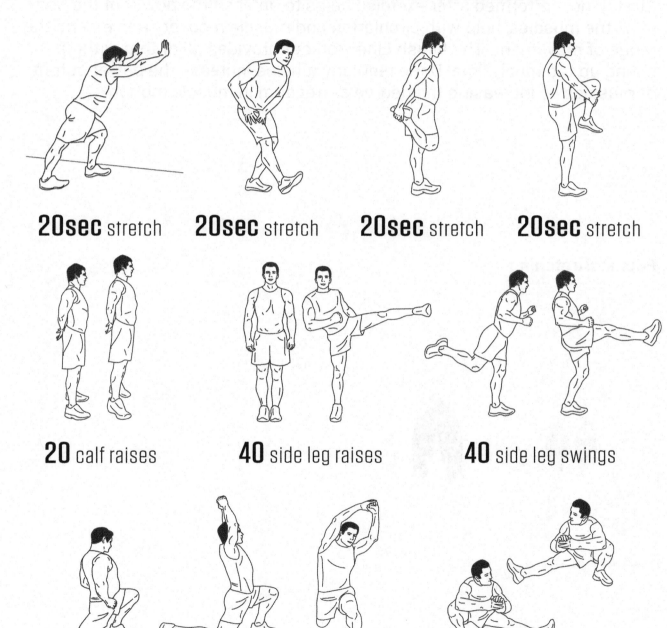

20sec stretch **20sec** stretch **20sec** stretch **20sec** stretch

20 calf raises **40** side leg raises **40** side leg swings

combo: 10sec each, then change legs **20** side-to-side lunges, toes up

49   Finish Line

Stretching, performed after exercise helps to unleash the power of the body, relax the muscles, help with circulation and muscle recovery and extend the range of movement. The Finish Line workout provides all of that without taking up too much time. Done regularly it helps increase the power output of muscles by increasing the degree of freedom in muscle motion.

Focus: Stretching

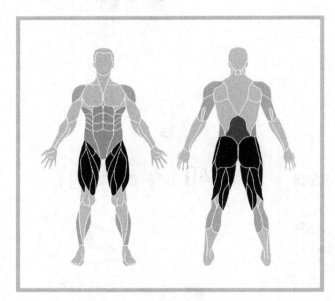

FINISH LINE

Go through the sequence:
once the move is done,
change sides and repeat again
for the same amount of time.

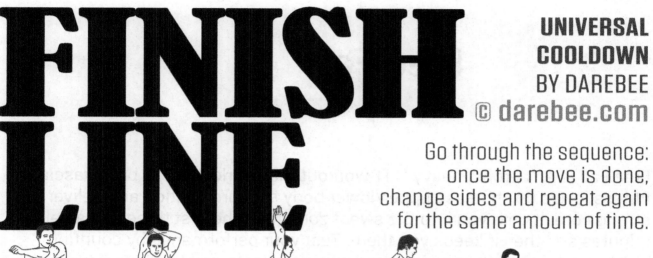
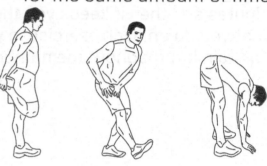

10sec stretch · **10sec** stretch · **10sec** reach · **10sec** stretch · **10sec** stretch · **10sec** reach

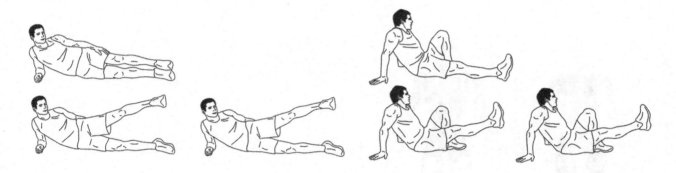

1min side leg raises + **30sec** hold · **1min** leg raises + **30sec** hold

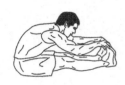
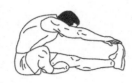
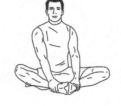
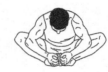
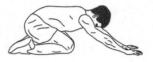

10sec reach · **10sec** reach · **10sec** stretch · **10sec** reach · **10sec** stretch

50   Free Fall

Free Fall is an aerobic-heavy HIIT workout that works hard to bring fascial fitness levels up, increase upper/lower body synchronization and deliver a strong core. It gets you into the sweat zone from the first three and a half minutes and then it keeps you there. Test your performance by counting what you do on each exercise in your first two sets and then see if you can maintain it throughout the number of sets you do.

Focus: High Burn, HIIT

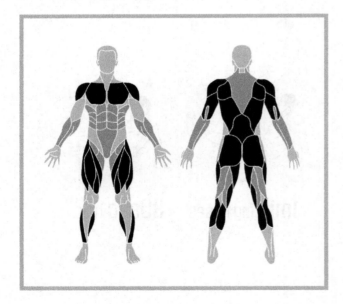

FREE FALL

DAREBEE `HIIT` WORKOUT
© **darebee.com**

Level I 3 sets
Level II 5 sets
Level III 7 sets
2 minutes rest between sets

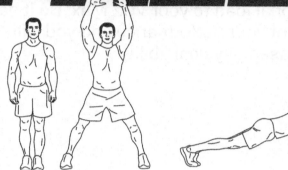 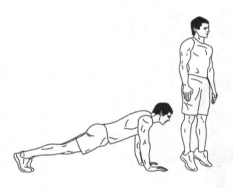 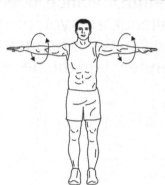

30sec jumping jacks   **30sec** basic burpees   **30sec** raised arm circles

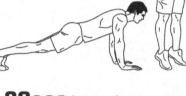

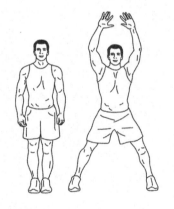

30sec jumping jacks   **30sec** basic burpees   **30sec** raised arm circles

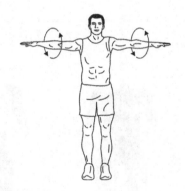

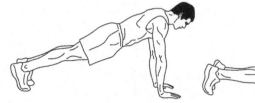 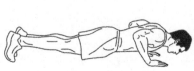 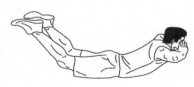

20sec push-up into back extension   +   **10sec** back extension hold

51 Fullbody Render

FullBody Render is a Level IV full-body workout that helps you develop strength, balance, coordination and endurance. Add EC as part of the challenge and you then have an additional load to your VO2 Max. Do it each time you want to push the boundaries of your performance and you will definitely feel the benefits of it in increased physical ability.

Focus: Strength & Tone

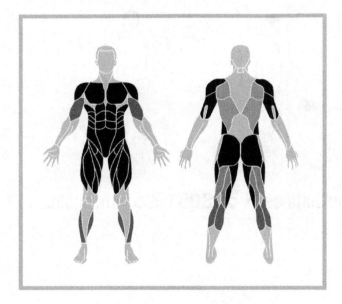

FULLBODY RENDER

DAREBEE WORKOUT © darebee.com

LEVEL I 3 sets **LEVEL II** 5 sets **LEVEL III** 7 sets **REST** up to 2 minutes

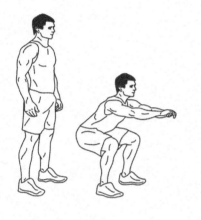

40 squats

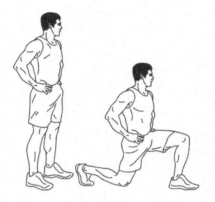

40 lunges

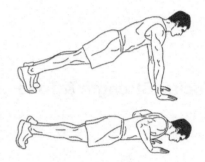

20 push-ups

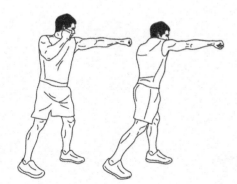

40 punches

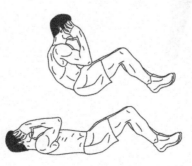

20 sit-ups

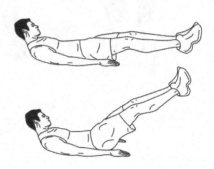

20 leg raises

52 Gambit

If you had really strong legs and a powerful core you would be able to synchronize your upper and lower body muscles in a way that would totally transform the way you move. The Gambit is there to make sure that your lower body and core are worked in a fashion that provides the foundation for just this kind of synchronization.

Focus: Strength & Tone

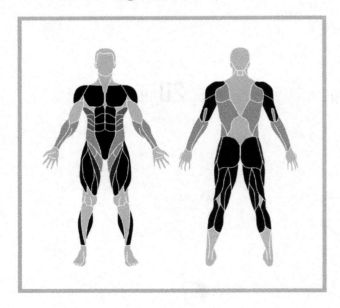

GAMBIT

DAREBEE WORKOUT © darebee.com

LEVEL I 3 sets **LEVEL II** 5 sets **LEVEL III** 7 sets **REST** up to 2 minutes

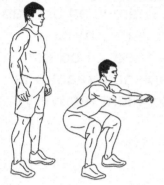

20 squats

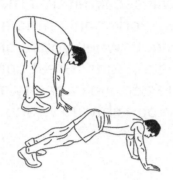

6 plank walk-outs

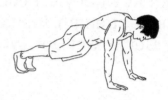

10-count plank hold

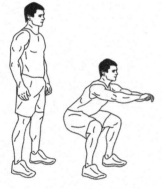

20 squats

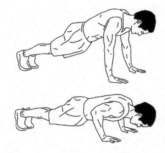

6 slow push-ups

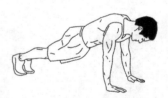

10-count plank hold

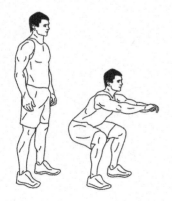

20 squats

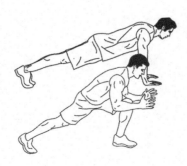

6 plank-into-lunges

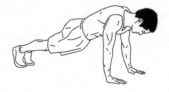

10-count plank hold

53   Heist

Some workouts are chosen and some workouts choose you. If you're doing The Heist workout you will see what that means. There is an overlap between anaerobic and aerobic work, concentric and eccentric muscle movement and isometric core work when you're already tired. Of course you know what you need for Heist, right? Great speed, splendid reactions, stamina, strength, focus, a little aerobic capacity and excellent recovery time. Get in. Get Out. What can possibly go wrong?

Focus: High Burn

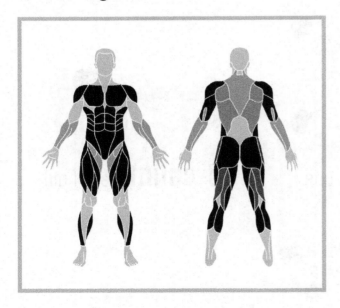

THE HEIST

DAREBEE WORKOUT
© darebee.com
LEVEL I 3 sets
LEVEL II 5 sets
LEVEL III 7 sets
REST up to 2 minutes

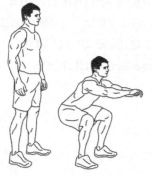
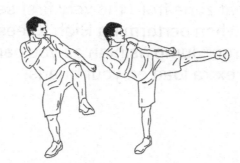
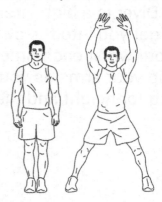

10combos: **1** squat + **2** double side kicks   **10** jumping jacks

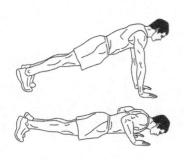
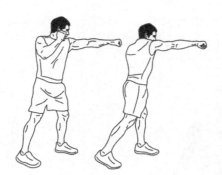
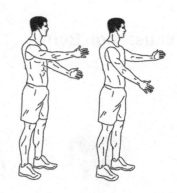

10combos: **1** push-ups + **4** punches   **10** scissor chops

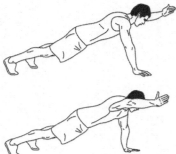
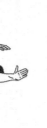
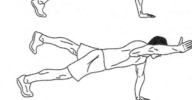

10 plank arm raises   **10** plank leg raises   **10** plank alt arm/ leg raises

54 Hell Diver

Hell Diver is a high intensity workout that will raise your body temperature and get you into the sweat zone from the very first set. Bring your knees up to your waist each time when performing High Knees and make sure you pump your arms as you run. Jump as high as you can in Basic Burpees, going for height and the extra load on your quads.

Focus: High Burn

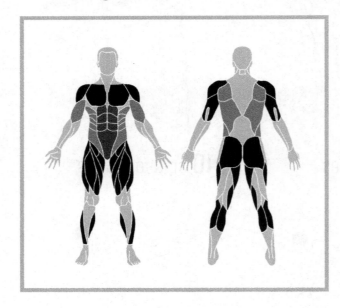

HELL DIVER

DAREBEE WORKOUT
© darebee.com
Level I 3 sets
Level II 5 sets
Level III 7 sets
2 minutes rest

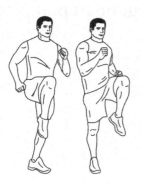

40 high knees

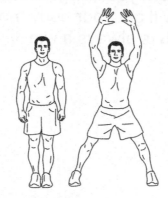

20 jumping jacks

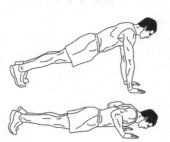

10 push-ups

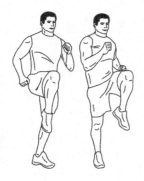

40 high knees

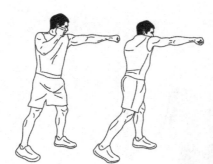

20 punches

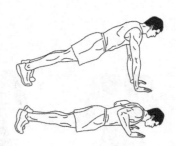

10 push-ups

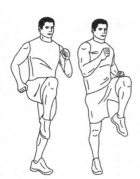

40 high knees

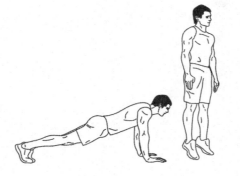

20 basic burpees

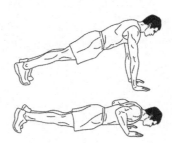

10 push-ups

55 Hell Raider

For days when you need a light, fast, energizing workout, Hell Raider delivers the goods. It won't burn your lungs, desiccate your body or make your muscles scream but it will get your body moving, your heart pumping and your lungs working which is always a win.

Focus: High Burn

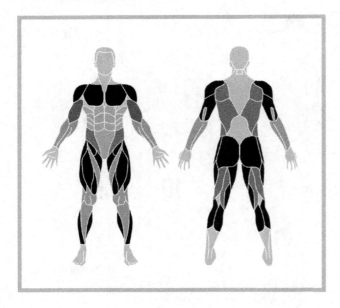

Hell Raider

"ONE HELL OF A RAID DAREBEE WORKOUT © darebee.com
LEVEL I 3 sets LEVEL II 5 sets LEVEL III 7 sets REST up to 2 minutes

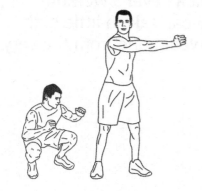

20 squat + side chop

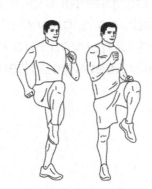

4combos: 10 high knees + **2** jump knee tucks

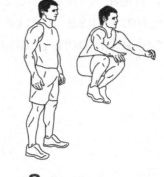

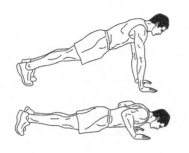

10 push-ups

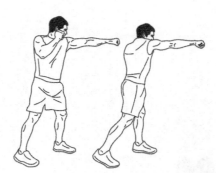

4combos: 10 punches + **2** hooks

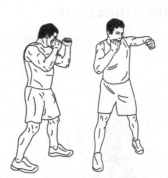

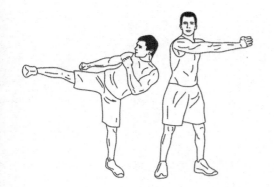

20 side kick + side chop

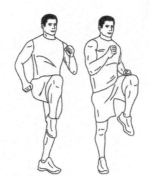

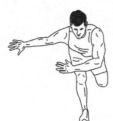

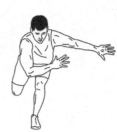

4combos: 10 high knees + **2** side-to-side jumps

56 Hightail

Hightail lives up to its name with a lot of march steps, high knees, jumping lunges and jump knee tucks. Despite all this it is still a Level 3 workout which means beginners can still do it, provided they can take a little high impact exercise. It is designed to get you into the sweat zone from the very first set and then, yeah it totally keeps you there.

Focus: High Burn

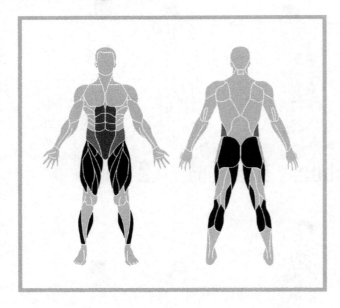

HIGHTAIL

DAREBEE WORKOUT © darebee.com

LEVEL I 3 sets **LEVEL II** 5 sets **LEVEL III** 7 sets **REST** up to 2 minutes

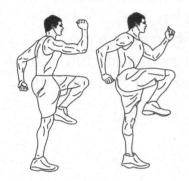

40 march steps

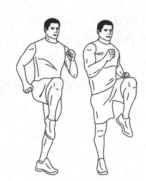

40 high knees

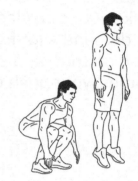

10 jump squats

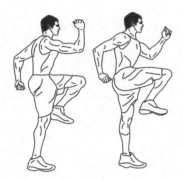

40 march steps

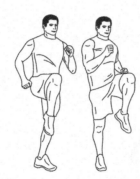

40 high knees

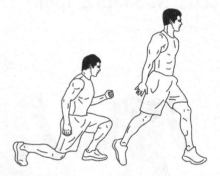

10 jumping lunges

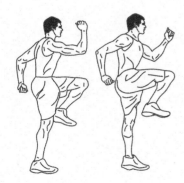

40 march steps

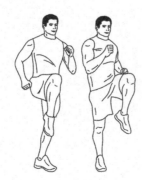

40 high knees

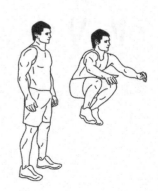

10 jump knee tucks

57 Hunter

If you had to hunt for your food you'd push yourself past every limit and overcome every barrier to catch your next meal. Hunter is a workout that will make your muscles work hard. It's not very heavy on aerobics but it does demand a lot from your muscles. Perform each exercise slowly, focusing on form and perfect execution. Keep your punches at chin height at all times, your push up deep, your body straight and your squats really deep.

Focus: Strength & Tone

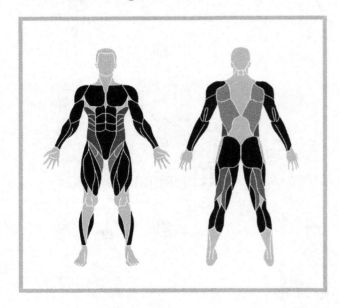

HUNTER

DAREBEE WORKOUT © darebee.com

LEVEL I 3 sets **LEVEL II** 5 sets **LEVEL III** 7 sets **REST** up to 2 minutes

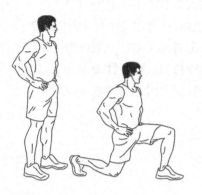

10 lunges

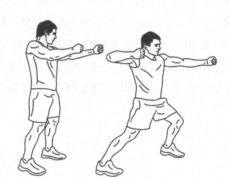

20 archer lunges

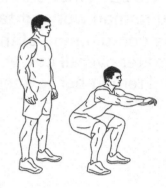

20 squats

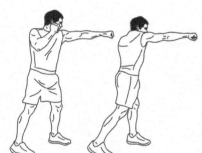

40 punches

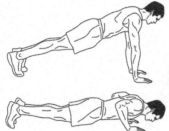

10 push-ups

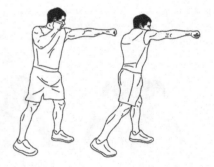

40 punches

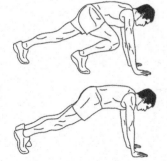

10 climbers

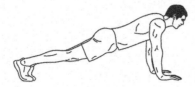

20-count plank

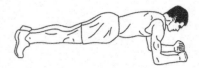

20-count elbow plank

58 Huntsman

Upper body strength requires a good strong core, pecs of steel and a strong lower back that connects the upper and lower parts of the trunk. The Huntsman workout takes you through a variety of push ups that require the coordination of the entire body, helping develop total body strength and greater overall power. Breathe in on the way down, exhale on the way up and remember to keep your body absolutely straight at all times.

Focus: Strength & Tone

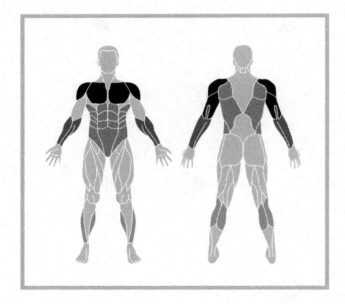

Huntsman

DAREBEE WORKOUT © darebee.com
LEVEL I 2 reps LEVEL II 4 reps LEVEL III 6 reps each
LEVEL I 3 sets LEVEL II 5 sets LEVEL III 7 sets
REST up to 2 minutes

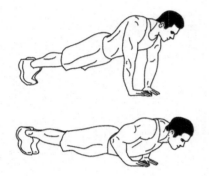

tricep push-ups

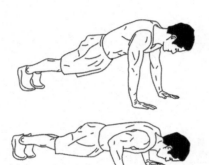

push-ups

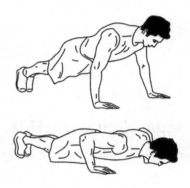

wide grip push-ups

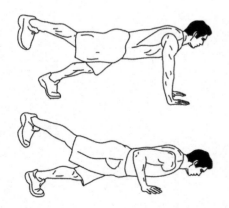

raised leg push-ups

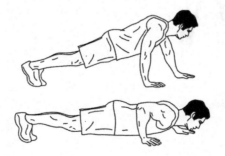

staggered push-ups

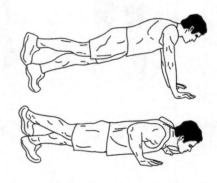

stacked push-ups

59 Inferno

Inferno is a Level 4 High Intensity Interval Training (HIIT) that places quite the load on the entire body and keeps it there for the duration of the workout. Make sure High Knees are performed by bringing the knee to the height of the waist and keep your body straight and your arms pumping while you are doing it. This is a high-burn, lots-of-sweat kind fo workout so be prepared to feel its effects.

Focus: High Burn, HIIT

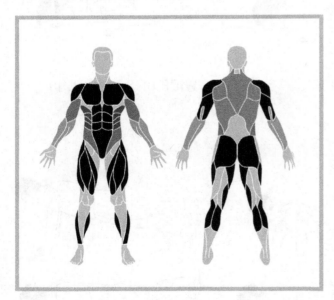

Inferno

DAREBEE HIIT WORKOUT © darebee.com

Level I 3 sets **Level II** 5 sets **Level III** 7 sets **REST** up to 2 minutes rest

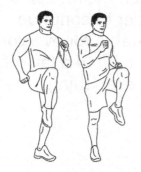 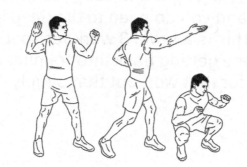 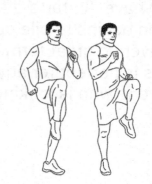

20sec high knees **20sec** knife hand strike + squat **20sec** high knees

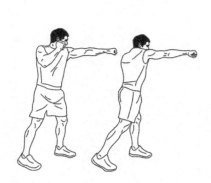 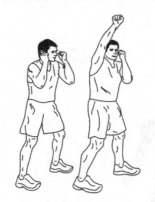 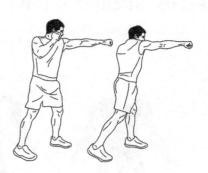

20sec punches **20sec** overhead punches **20sec** punches

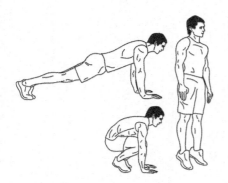 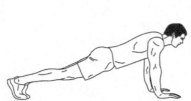 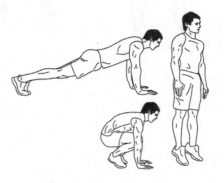

20sec basic burpees **20sec** plank hold **20sec** basic burpees

60   Initiation

Initiation is a total body workout that recruits every major muscle group you have. It starts off feeling light and easy but the load on the muscles soon begins to pile up and you do need to dig deep in order to continue delivering great form. This is a Level 3 workout so it's suitable for everyone. This is perfect for anyone getting back into training after a bit of a lay off or anyone who is looking for that workout that simply does everything.

Focus: Strength & Tone

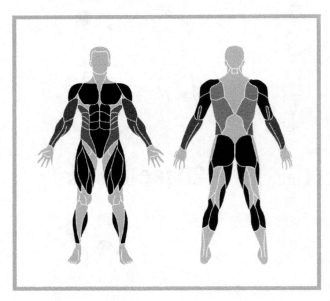

INITIATION

DAREBEE WORKOUT © darebee.com

LEVEL I 3 sets **LEVEL II** 5 sets **LEVEL III** 7 sets **REST** up to 2 minutes

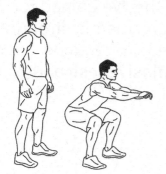

40 squats

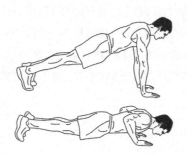

5 push-ups

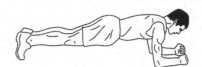

20-count elbow plank

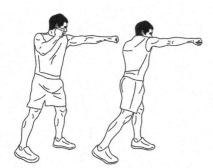

40 punches

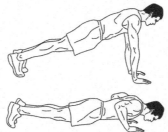

5 push-ups

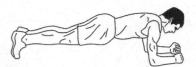

20-count elbow plank

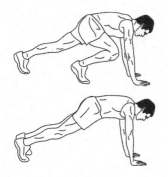

40 climbers

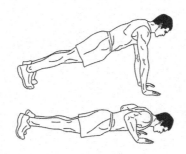

5 push-ups

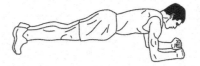

20-count elbow plank

61 Iron Bar

Tendons are the cable anchors that stabilize our muscles. Tendons require a lot of work to get strong, but hold onto the strength they've gained for long times of inactivity if they have to. Powerful tendons means strong, stable muscles. The Iron Bar workout is there to make your tendons hard and strong. It'll help increase stability, speed, explosiveness and coordination. It delivers, in short, greater body control.

Focus: Stretching

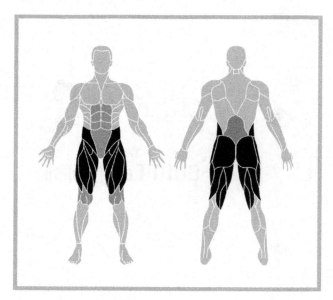

iron bar

TENDON STRENGTH
DAREBEE WORKOUT © darebee.com

Change legs after each sequence
and repeat it again. Keep your leg off the floor
throughout the sequence. Perfect post workout.

SEQUENCE 1

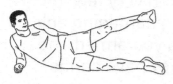

15-count hold

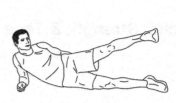

15 side leg raises

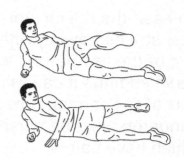

15 straight leg swings

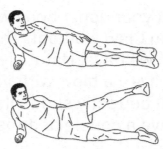

15 fast kicks

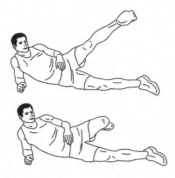

15 slow kicks

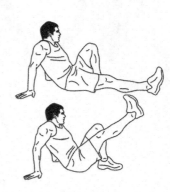

15-count hold

SEQUENCE 2

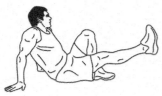

15-count hold

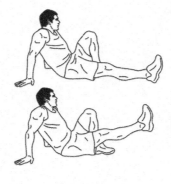

15 leg raises

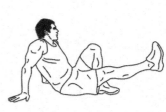

15 high leg raises

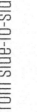

15 move from side-to-side

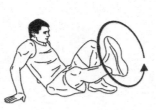

15 circles

15-count hold

62   Iron Claw

Unleash the tiger in you and get your upper body working and your palm heel strikes flowing with the Iron Claw workout. The heel of the palm is one of the few natural weapons we have. Naturally hard with very few nerve endings it can take (or deliver) a blow without risking damaging any part of it. Learning how to use it correctly suddenly makes you armed and dangerous just because you have a couple of arms and they have hands which have palms.

Focus: Strength & Tone

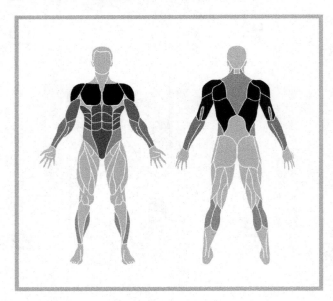

IronClaw

DAREBEE WORKOUT © darebee.com

LEVEL I 3 sets **LEVEL II** 4 sets **LEVEL III** 5 sets **REST** up to 2 minutes

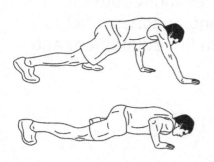 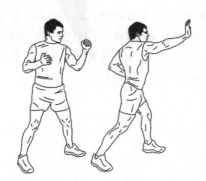 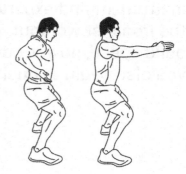

10 dragon push-up   **10** palm strikes   **10** squat hold rows

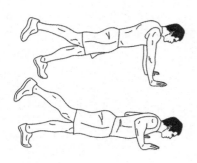 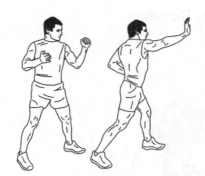 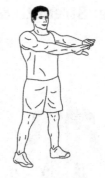

10 raised leg push-ups   **10** palm strikes   **20-count** raised arm hold

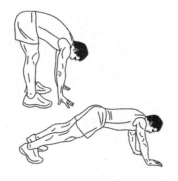 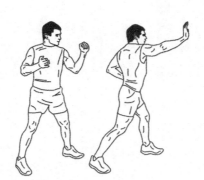 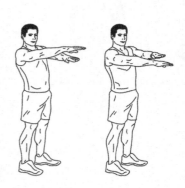

10 plank walk-outs   **10** palm strikes   **20** scissors

63 Iron Fist

Sharpen up your combat skills, hone your body into a finely-tuned instrument and experience the power of having it under your control with the Iron Fist workout. Using a combination of kicks and punches it helps build speed, power, coordination and stability. Add the EC requirement and you also begin to push your VO2 Max capacity.

Focus: Strength & Tone, Combat

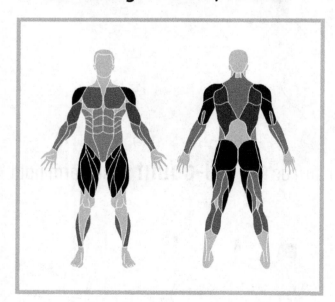

IRON FIST

DAREBEE WORKOUT © darebee.com

Level I 3 sets **Level II** 5 sets **Level III** 7 sets **REST** up to 2 minutes rest

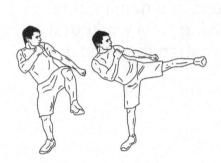

20 side kicks

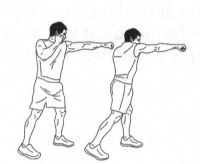

20 jab + cross

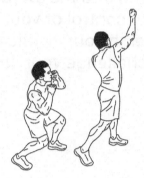

20 uppercuts

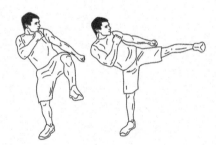

20 side kicks

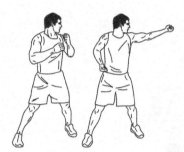

20 backfists

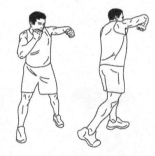

20 hooks

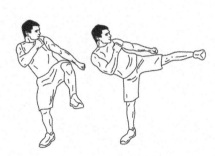

20 side kicks

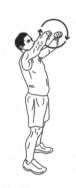

20 speed bag punches

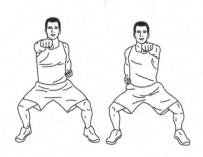

100 squat hold punches

64 Iron Maiden

Iron Maiden is a total body core strength and endurance workout that will get you into the sweat zone within minutes of starting. Great for gaining better control of your body, activating muscle groups and gaining more power in your physical performance. If you are looking for a workout that will challenge your strength, endurance and coordination then this is the one.

Focus: Strength & Tone

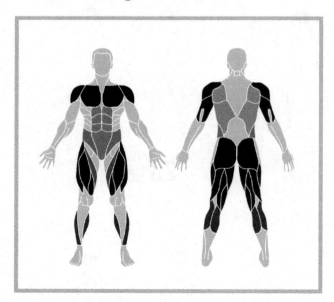

IRON MAIDEN

DAREBEE WORKOUT © darebee.com

LEVEL I 3 sets **LEVEL II** 4 sets **LEVEL III** 5 sets **REST** up to 2 minutes

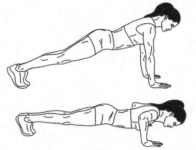

40 squats

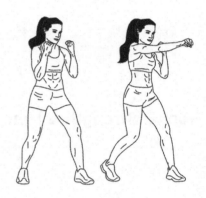

10 push-ups

40 punches

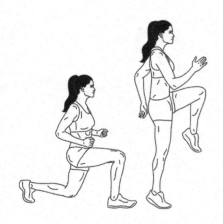

40 lunge step-ups

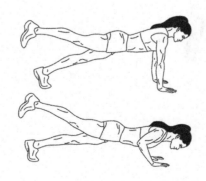

10 raised leg push-ups

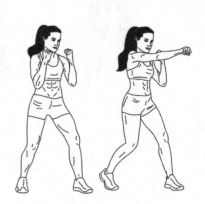

40 punches

65 Kamikaze

Sometimes the simplicity of a workout is in direct proportion to the magnitude of its level of difficulty and the Kamikaze workout proves the rule. Five simple exercises in sequence push your muscles to the very limit, recruiting additional muscle groups to help compensate for the ever increasing load that is brought to bear. The result is a Level 5 difficulty workout that will help you get strong ... very, very strong.

Focus: Strength & Tone

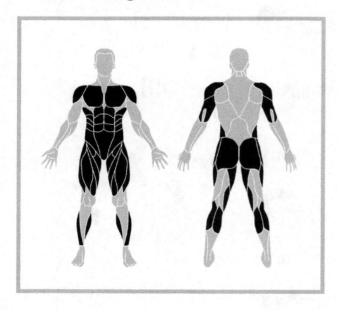

KAMIKAZE

DAREBEE WORKOUT © darebee.com
LEVEL I 3 sets LEVEL II 4 sets LEVEL III 5 sets
2 minutes rest between sets

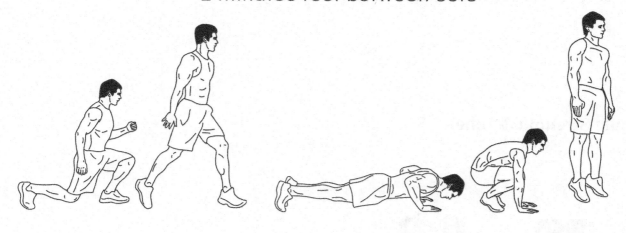

30 jumping lunges   **30** burpees

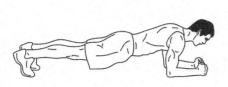 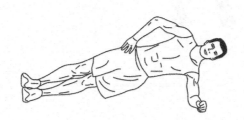 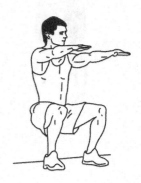

1min elbow plank   **1min** side elbow plank   **1min** wall sit

66 King of the Hill

King of the Hill is the kind of workout that takes you through a Climb, Take Over and then Hold the "Hill" workout that works on your attributes of strength, power and stability by training the body's major muscles. There is a strong core training component here which will be truly beneficial to your performance in other sports and workouts. This is not an overly taxing workout from an aerobic performance point of view but it will definitely stretch you a little where your muscular strength is concerned.

Focus: Strength & Tone

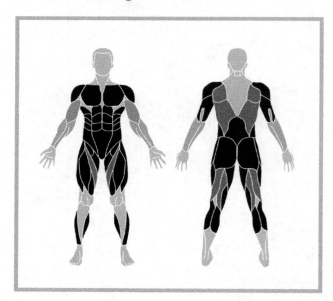

KING OF THE HILL

DAREBEE WORKOUT
ⓒ **darebee.com**
LEVEL I 3 sets
LEVEL II 5 sets
LEVEL III 7 sets
REST up to 2 minutes

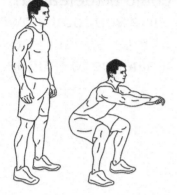
20 squats

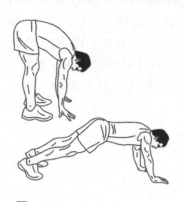
5 plank walk-outs

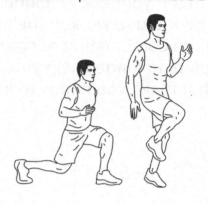
20 lunge step-ups

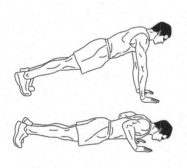
5 push-ups

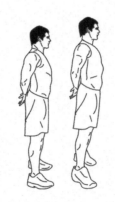
20 calf raises

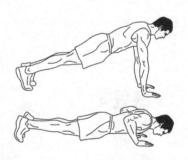
5 push-ups

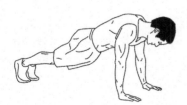
20-count plank

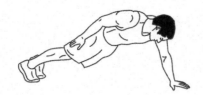
20-count one-arm plank

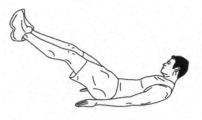
20-count raised leg hold

67 Kitsune

What if your body weighed almost nothing and gravity could be defeated? The Kitsune workout helps you learn to move your body like you totally own it. Its combination of combat moves, jump knee tucks, lunges, squats and jumping lunges help your muscles develop the kind of resilience to fatigue that make you happy to live inside your body.

Focus: High Burn

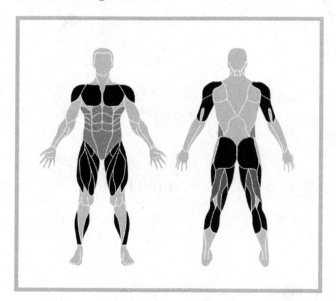

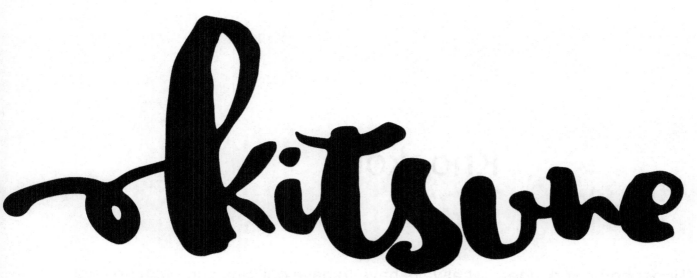

kitsune

DAREBEE WORKOUT © darebee.com

LEVEL I 3 sets **LEVEL II** 5 sets **LEVEL III** 7 sets **REST** up to 2 minutes

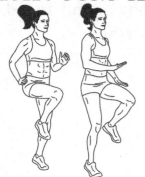

20 high knees

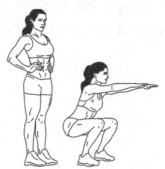

20 squats

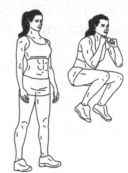

4 jump knee tucks

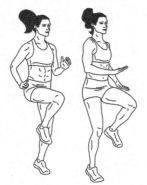

20 high knees

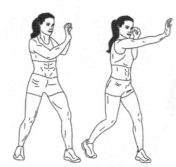

20 palm strikes

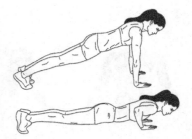

4 push-ups

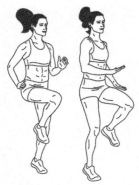

20 high knees

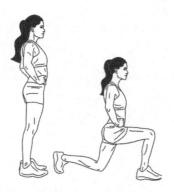

20 lunges

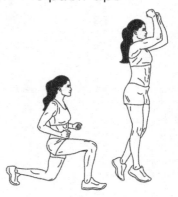

4 jumping lunges

68 Knockout

Upper body work does not always have to have pull ups and push ups nor does it require weights. A dynamic approach that employs shadow boxing moves and precise martial arts techniques pushes the muscles to work in both concentric and eccentric ways increasing effective power and speed. Don't spare yourself, the Knockout workout is here to help you.

Focus: Strength & Tone, Combat

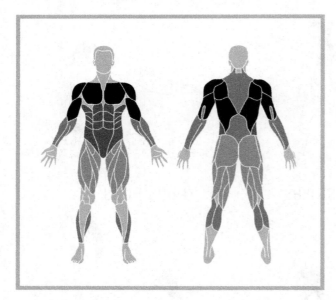

KNOCKOUT

DAREBEE WORKOUT © darebee.com

LEVEL I 3 sets **LEVEL II** 5 sets **LEVEL III** 7 sets **REST** up to 2 minutes

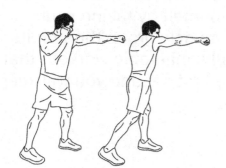

40 jab + cross

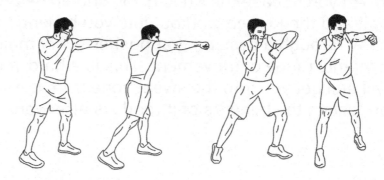

20combos jab + cross + elbow strike + hook

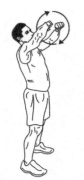

40 speed bag punches

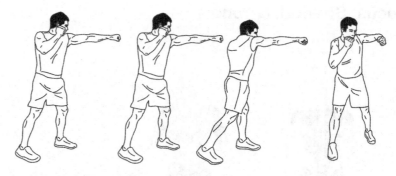

20combos jab + jab + cross + hook

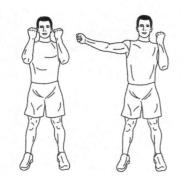

40 side-to-side backfists

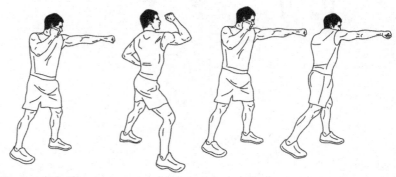

20combos jab + elbow strike + jab + cross

69 Kraken

When you release the Kraken you should be prepared to feel every moment of it and the Kraken workout lets you be kind to yourself by taking your body through a session that pushes every major muscle group through its dynamic range of movement. This is a hard, mostly anaerobic workout that will still get you into the sweat zone from the very first set and you will keep on feeling the benefits of it for days afterward.

Focus: Strength & Tone

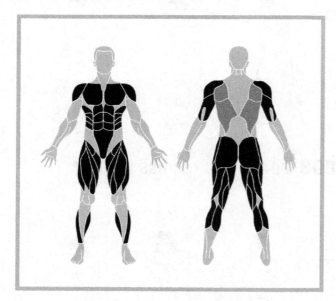

RELEASE THE
KRAKEN

DAREBEE WORKOUT © darebee.com

LEVEL I 3 sets **LEVEL II** 5 sets **LEVEL III** 7 sets **REST** up to 2 minutes

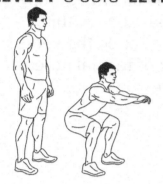

20 squats

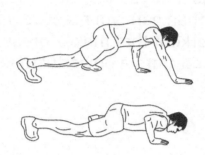

6 dragon push-ups

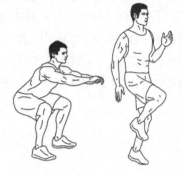

20 squats step-ups

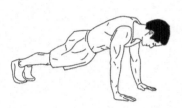

20-count plank

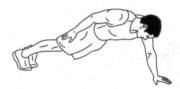

20-count one arm plank

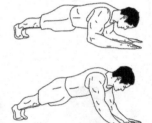

6 tricep extensions

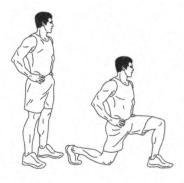

20 lunges

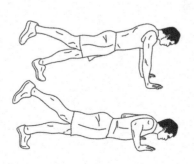

6 raised leg push-ups

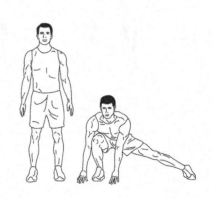

20 deep side lunges

70 Launch Codes

Go ballistic with the Launch Codes workout. Whether you are throwing punches in midair or are throwing your body through the air with Jump Knee-Tucks the sure thing is that you will be in the sweat zone within minutes and you will more than earn your recovery break once the set is over. This is a total body workout that makes great use of fascial fitness exercises to help turn the body into a powerful machine.

Focus: Strength & Tone

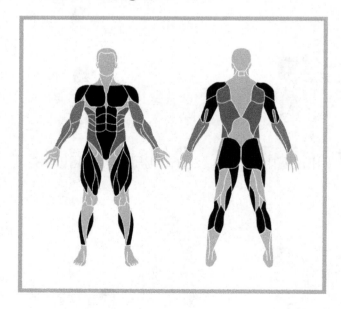

LAUNCH CODES

DAREBEE WORKOUT
© darebee.com
LEVEL I 3 sets
LEVEL II 5 sets
LEVEL III 7 sets
REST up to 2 minutes

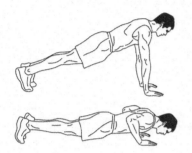

5 push-ups

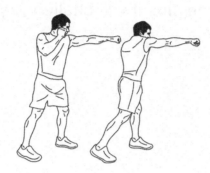

30 punches

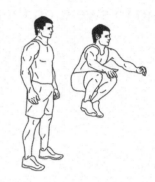

5 jump knee-tucks

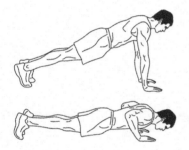

5 push-ups

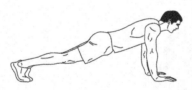

30-count plank

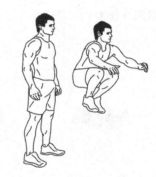

5 jump knee-tucks

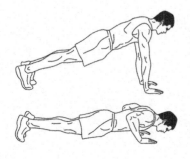

5 push-ups

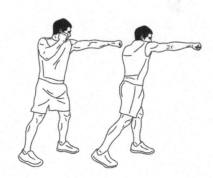

30 punches

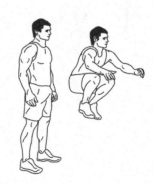

5 jump knee-tucks

71 Live Wire

Livewire is a fast-flowing, high burn workout that's accessible and yet delivers a very targeted, total body training experience. You know you're going to sweat on this one plus it will challenge your VO2 Max level.

Focus: High Burn

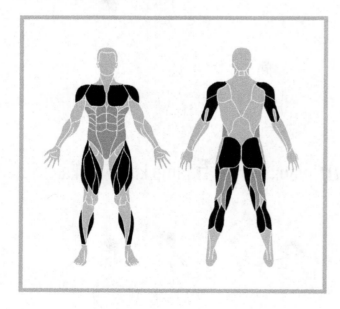

LIVE WIRE

DAREBEE WORKOUT © darebee.com

LEVEL I 3 sets **LEVEL II** 5 sets **LEVEL III** 7 sets **REST** up to 2 minutes

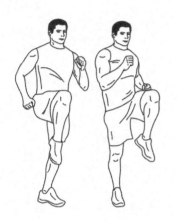

60 high knees

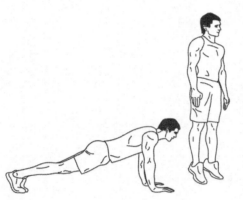

10 basic burpee w/jump

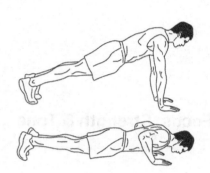

10 push-ups

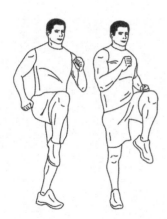

60 high knees

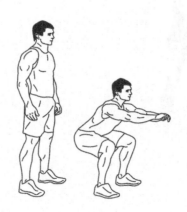

10 squats

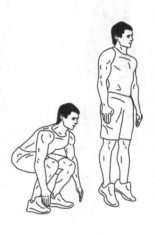

10 jump squats

72 Lumberjack

Arguably nothing gets you quite as strong as cutting down trees with an ax. That's not very environmentally friendly however so the Lumberjack workout is the next best thing. In a set of nine exercise routines it loads all the major muscle groups in the body providing a total strength workout that will help you develop stronger, more powerful muscles.

Focus: Strength & Tone

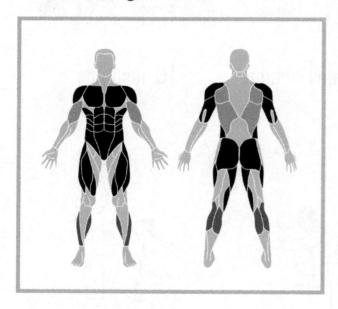

LUMBERJACK

DAREBEE WORKOUT © darebee.com

LEVEL I 3 sets **LEVEL II** 5 sets **LEVEL III** 7 sets **REST** up to 2 minutes

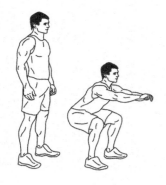
20 lunges

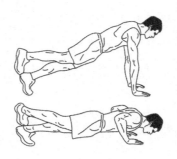
10 stacked push-ups

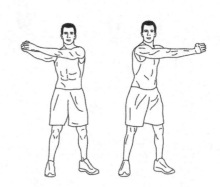
40 side-to-side chops

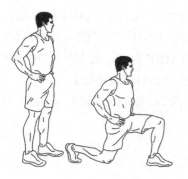
20 slow climbers

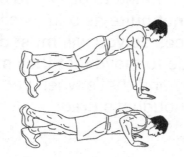
10 stacked push-ups

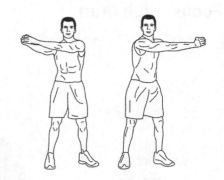
40 side-to-side chops

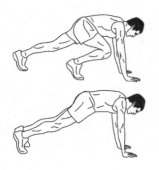
20 squats

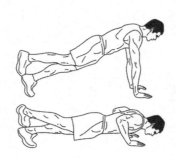
10 stacked push-ups

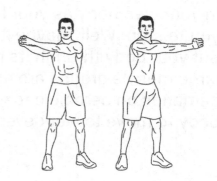
40 side-to-side chops

73 Mutiny

The Mutiny workout is inspired by the frenetic energy of a mutiny but its push on aerobic capacity and total body strength may well signal a mutiny in your own body as your legs refuse to obey you and your lungs scream at you to stop. Well, maybe it's not quite as bad as all that but it is designed to put your body through its paces so you will most definitely feel it. Whenever large muscle groups are made to move fast they make tremendous demands on aerobic capacity and that's when you start to condition your body to move to work even though it's tired.

Focus: High Burn

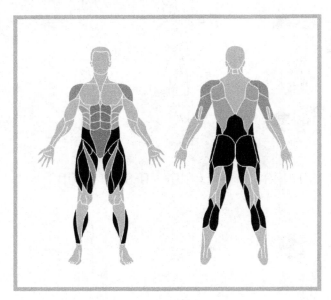

MUTINY

DAREBEE WORKOUT © darebee.com

LEVEL I 3 sets **LEVEL II** 5 sets **LEVEL III** 7 sets **REST** up to 2 minutes

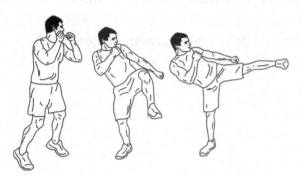

20 bounce, bounce + side kick

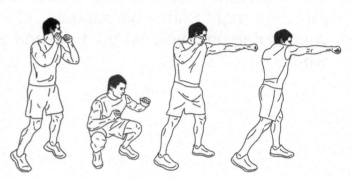

20 bounce, bounce + squat + jab + cross

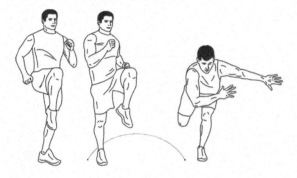

4 combos: 10 high knees + **1** jump to the side

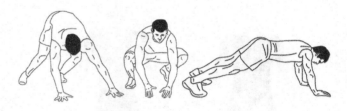

4 combos: 1 ape hop + **1** plank walk-out

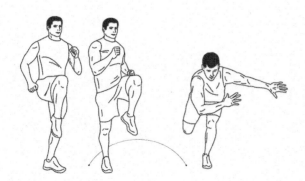

4 combos: 10 high knees + **1** jump to the side

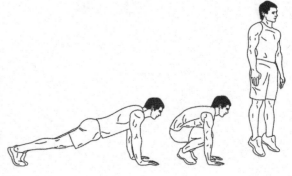

4 basic burpees with a jump

74　Night Shift

You don't need to be working a night shift to do the Night Shift workout but if you are then you could do it, provided you have a little bit of time and just a tiny amount of space. Designed to help you maintain strength and muscle tone, the Night Shift workout uses all the major muscle groups to keep you revving until you get the time and energy for an even more energetic workout.

Focus: Strength & Tone

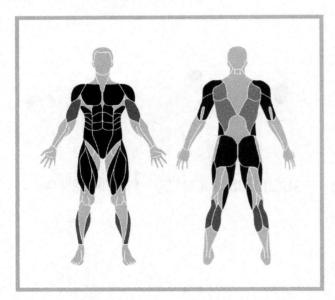

NIGHT SHIFT

DAREBEE WORKOUT © darebee.com

LEVEL I 3 sets **LEVEL II** 5 sets **LEVEL III** 7 sets **REST** up to 2 minutes

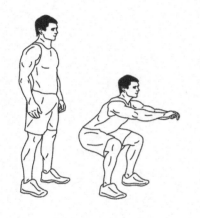

20 squats

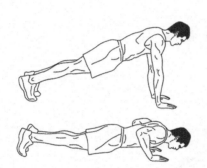

20 push-ups

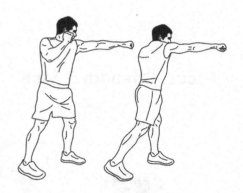

20 punches

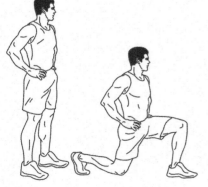

20 lunges

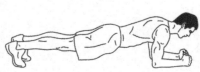

20sec plank

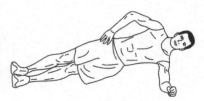

40sec side plank

75 No Capes

No Capes may be safer for superhero types but the No Capes workout pulls no punches when it comes to making your body work hard. It gets you in the sweat zone really fast and keeps you there until the very end. No Capes works almost every major muscle group and maintains the load throughout the workout.

Focus: Strength & Tone

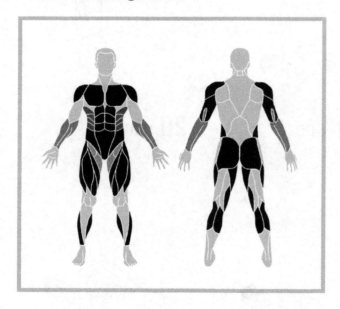

N⊘ CAPES

DAREBEE WORKOUT © darebee.com

LEVEL I 3 sets **LEVEL II** 5 sets **LEVEL III** 7 sets **REST** up to 2 minutes

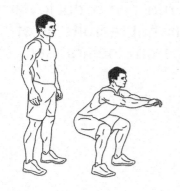

20 squats

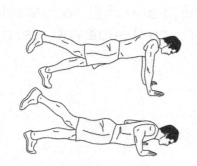

10 raised leg push-ups

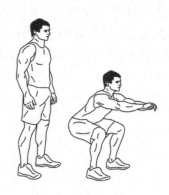

20 squats

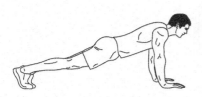

10-count plank

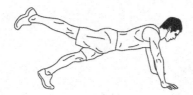

10-count raised leg plank

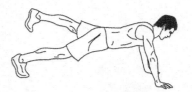

10-count raised leg plank

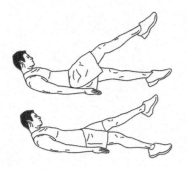

10 flutter kicks

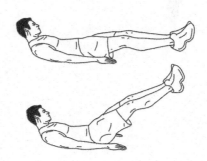

10 leg raises

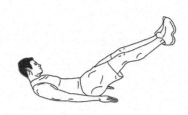

10-count raised leg hold

76 Off the Grid

Off The Grid is the kind of workout that prepares you for what happens when the Zombie Apocalypse arrives and you have to run, climb, duck, carry heavy stuff and fight. It's a high-burn full body workout that recruits all of the major muscle groups for a challenge you feel right from the first set.

Focus: High Burn

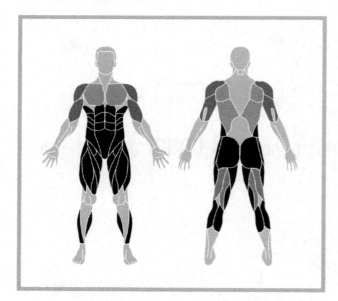

OFF THE GRID

DAREBEE WORKOUT © darebee.com

LEVEL I 3 sets **LEVEL II** 5 sets **LEVEL III** 7 sets **REST** up to 2 minutes

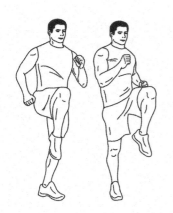

40 high knees

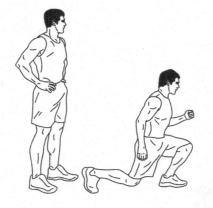

20 lunges

20sec elbow plank

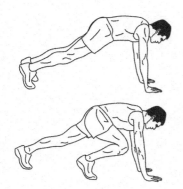

20 climbers

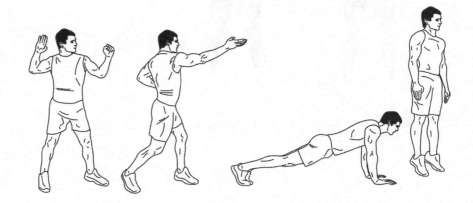

40 knife hand strikes

20 basic burpees

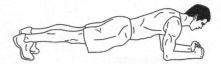

77   One Punch

The One Punch workout is an anaerobic, fast-paced strength and power-orientated workout. It won't feel like much doing the first set or even the second but as your muscle temperature rises and the on-board ATP stores are depleted you are going to feel the burn. Your mission is to maintain the pace throughout so as your muscles get more tired your pace and output do not slacken.

Focus: Strength & Tone

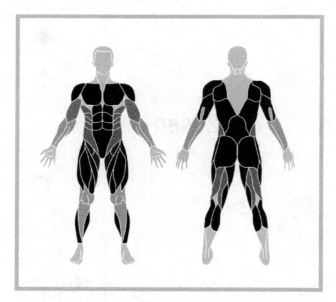

ONE PUNCH

DAREBEE TRIBUTE WORKOUT © darebee.com

10 sets or as many as you can do | up to 2 minutes rest between sets

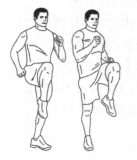 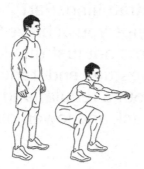 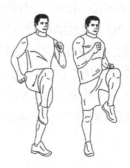 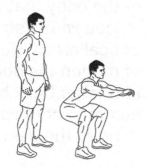

10 high knees   **5** squats   **10** high knees   **5** squats

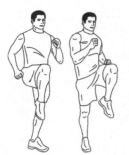 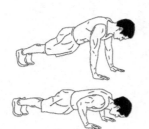 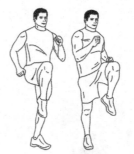 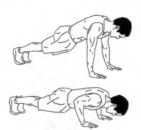

10 high knees   **5** push-ups   **10** high knees   **5** push-ups

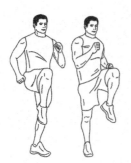 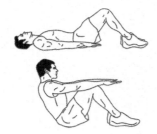 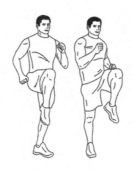 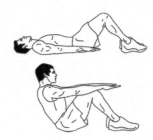

10 high knees   **5** sit-ups   **10** high knees   **5** sit-ups

The adductors, lower back and the psoas are amongst the components of the body that are overlooked when stretching. Part 2 comes to the rescue with a stretching routine that helps you achieve flexibility in these critical areas. How supple you are affects not just the degrees of freedom of motion the body achieves but also posture, endurance, core strength and lower back health. Make this workout a regular and many of the most common complaints regarding lower back and lower joints pain will be a thing of the past.

Focus: Stretching

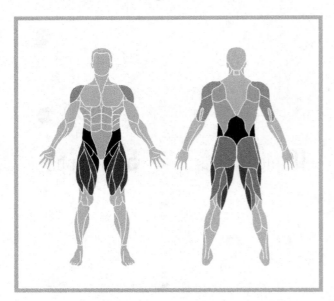

PART 2

DAREBEE POST-WORKOUT STRETCHING © darebee.com
30 seconds = 15 seconds per side / leg

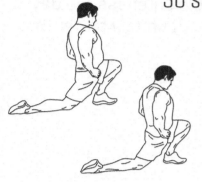

1. lunge stretches

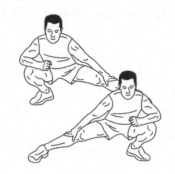

2. side-to-side lunges

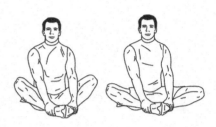

3. butterfly stretches

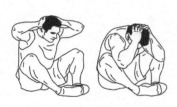

4. back stretches

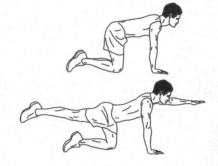

5. opposite arm / leg raises

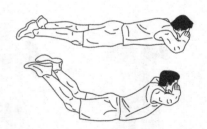

6. back extensions

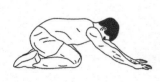

7. stretch

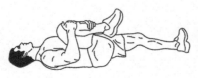

8. stretch

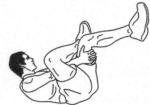

9. stretch

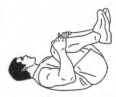

10. stretch

79 Plan B

A Plan B workout is there for when there is no plan A. This is a 'gentle' workout. It won't push you to the limits, you won't be reduced to swearing under your breath and there won't even be much muscle soreness the day after, but it will still give you a decent workout which is definitely better than none.

Focus: Strength & Tone

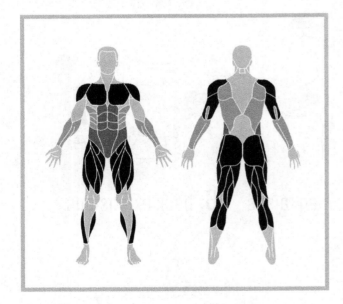

PLAN B

DAREBEE WORKOUT © darebee.com

LEVEL I 3 sets **LEVEL II** 5 sets **LEVEL III** 7 sets **REST** up to 2 minutes

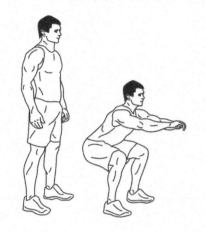

20 squats

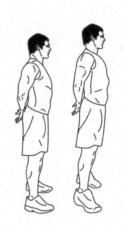

20 calf raises

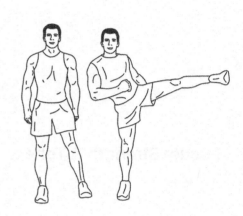

20 side leg raises

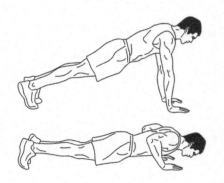

10 push-ups

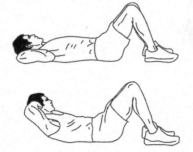

10 crunches

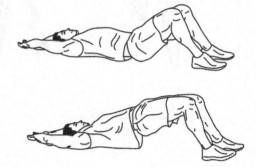

10 bridges

80	# Power Mode

Strength is the ability of the muscles to perform work at a high intensity consistently and it is build, over time, by making muscle groups work under load on the entire muscle fiber. This is a workout that is performed deliberately and with focus. Attention is paid to technique so that form is maintained. You won't get out of breath but you will work up a sweat.

Focus: Strength & Tone

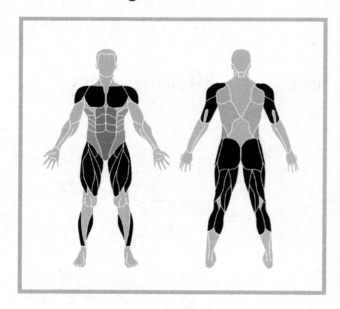

POWER MODE

DAREBEE WORKOUT © darebee.com

LEVEL I 3 sets **LEVEL II** 5 sets **LEVEL III** 7 sets **REST** up to 2 minutes

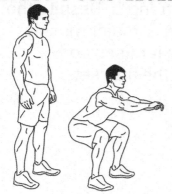

20 squats

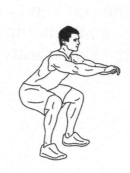

20-count squat hold

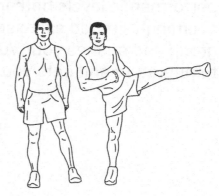

20 side leg raises

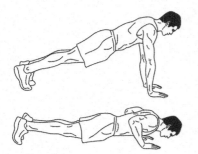

10 push-ups

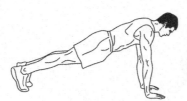

10-count plank

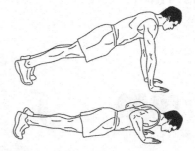

10 push-ups

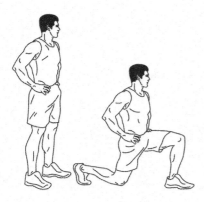

20 lunges

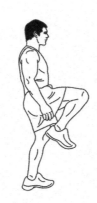

20-count balance hold

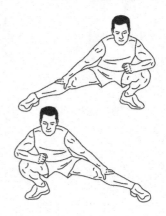

20 side lunges

81 Power Run

Power Run uses two seemingly simple exercises to help you push your performance levels both in terms of endurance and strength. Despite the seemingly limited exercise set the workout targets every major muscle group and pushes your VO2 Max ability to the limit as it raises body temperature and gets you into the sweat zone within the first set.

Focus: High Burn

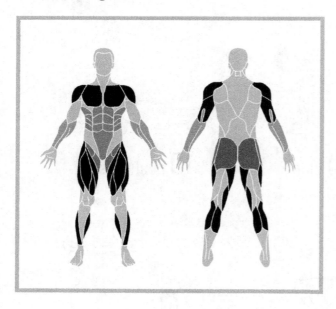

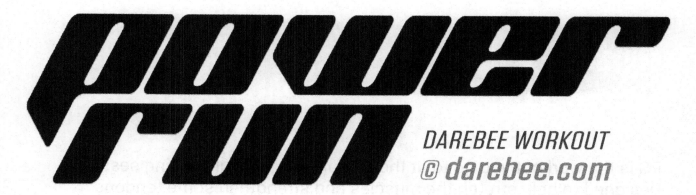

power run

DAREBEE WORKOUT
© darebee.com

LEVEL I 3 sets **LEVEL II** 5 sets **LEVEL III** 7 sets **REST** up to 2 minutes

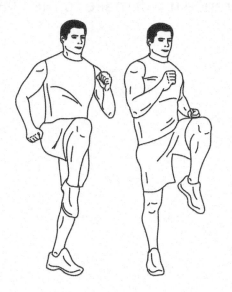

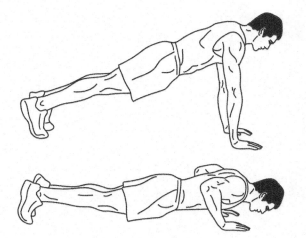

20 high knees

2 push-ups

20 high knees

2 push-ups

20 high knees

2 push-ups

20 high knees

2 push-ups

20 high knees

2 push-ups

20 high knees

2 push-ups

done

82   P. S.

PS is the workout you go to at the end of each of your training sessions. Designed to help stretch the muscles and strengthen some tendons it also delivers the kind of concentrated, lower body muscle tone work that you know is helping you get more from your body's strength and natural athleticism. Make this one of the constants in your after-workout routine and you will be surprised by the difference it will make to the way you move your body.

Focus: Stretching

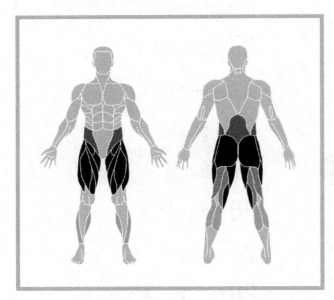

P.S.

DAREBEE
POST-WORKOUT
© darebee.com

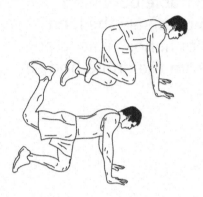 **40** leg extensions

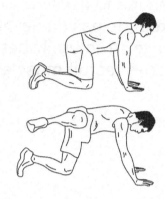 **40** side leg extensions

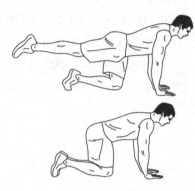 **40** straight leg extensions

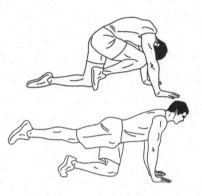 **40** knee in extensions

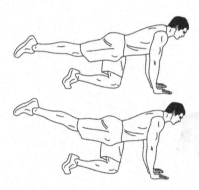 **40** extended swings

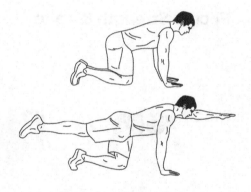 **40** alt arm / leg raises

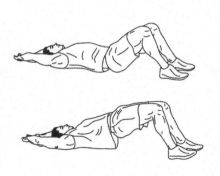 **10** bridges

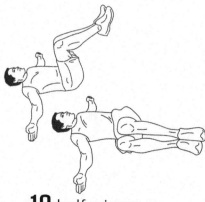 **10** half wipers

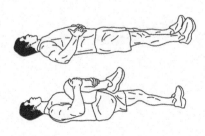 **10** knee hugs

83 Punch Out

It takes strength, speed and stamina to develop sustainable punching power and the Punch Out! workout helps you develop precisely the kind of power you need in order to have structurally better punches. This is an upper body workout, though it does recruit muscles from the entire body in order to power those punches.

Focus: Strength & Tone

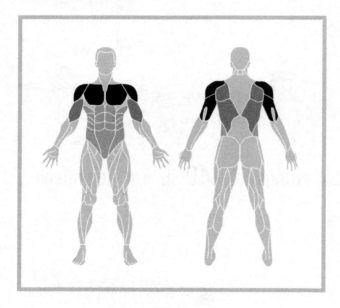

PUNCH OUT!

DAREBEE WORKOUT © darebee.com

LEVEL I 3 sets **LEVEL II** 5 sets **LEVEL III** 7 sets **REST** up to 2 minutes

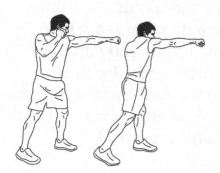

20 punches

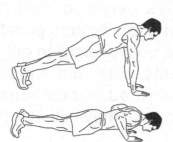

6 push-ups

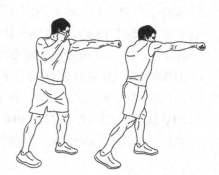

20 punches

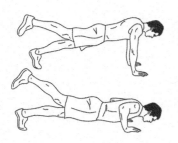

6 raised leg push-ups

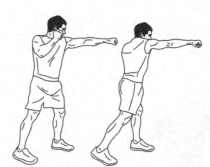

20 punches

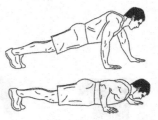

6 staggered push-ups

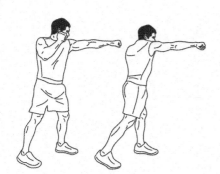

20 punches

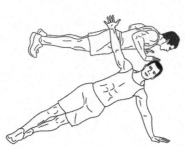

6 push-up + rotation

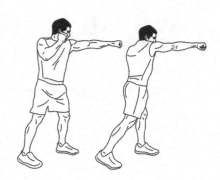

20 punches

84 Push-Up Massacre

Civilization has only been made possible because of our upper body strength and our ability to dexterously use our arms and hands. Push-ups are a great way to use the body's weight to challenge its muscles. They train all the major abdominal muscle groups plus the upper body and enable us to take on our whole body weight in our own hands. Push-Up Massacre, as the name suggests, puts your arms to the test by forcing your body to work in different muscle-loading positions. Your arms may scream a little in the process but ultimately they will just thank you for it!

Focus: Strength & Tone

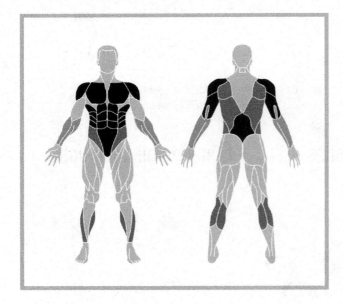

push-up massacre

LEVEL I 3 sets
LEVEL II 4 sets
LEVEL III 5 sets
2 minutes rest

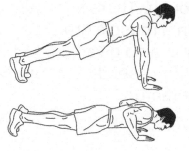

6 classic push-ups

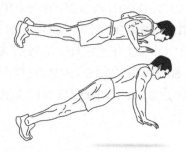

6 power push-ups

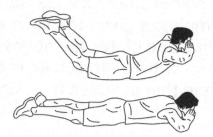

4 back extensions

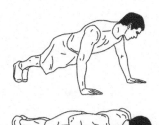
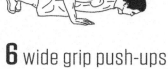

6 wide grip push-ups

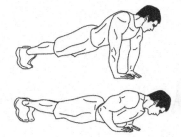

6 close grip push-ups

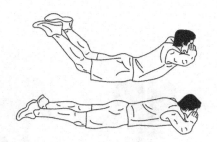

4 back extensions

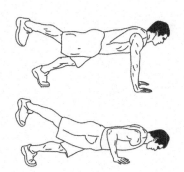

6 raised leg push-ups

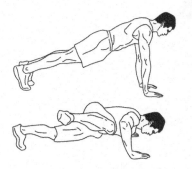

6 side crunch push-ups

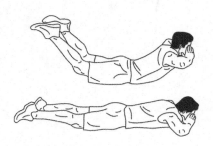

4 back extensions

85 Ragnarok

Ragnarok is a strength workout that takes the body through slow, deep moves, executed in perfect form to slowly but steadily load the muscles so that they begin to feel the need to adapt. This is a deceptive-looking workout where the exercises themselves look easy enough. There is some emphasis given to the core as well as the four abdominal muscle groups. Hips and glutes are not overlooked and the lower body is also given a good workout. The trick here is to slow things down, rather than speed them up (and that includes the side kicks) adding to the fatigue factor.

Focus: Strength & Tone

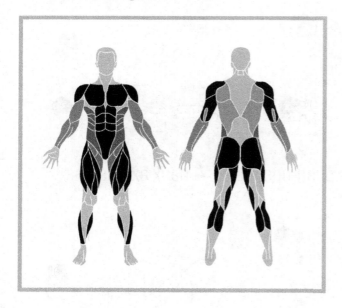

RAGNARÖK

DAREBEE WORKOUT © darebee.com

Level I 3 sets **Level II** 5 sets **Level III** 7 sets **REST** up to 2 minutes rest

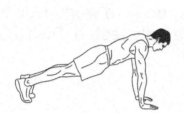

20 push-ups

20-count plank hold

20 jab + cross

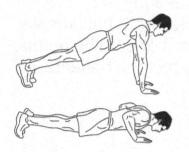

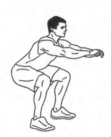

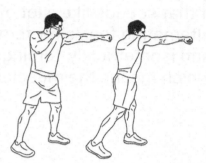

20 squats

20-count squat hold

20 side kicks

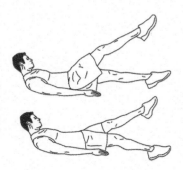

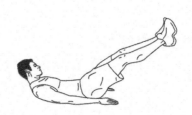

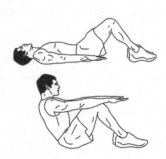

20 flutter kicks

20-count raised leg hold

20 sit-ups

86 Reboot

Reboot your body, mind and spirit with the Reboot workout designed to get you moving, your arms and legs pumping and your heart thumping. If that sounds like a lot of hard work it is because it is exactly that. The alternating fast/slow tempo segments work the muscles both ballistically and isometrically, forcing your body to work even when it should be resting which means the muscles are truly tested. Dive in and feel the benefits.

Focus: High Burn

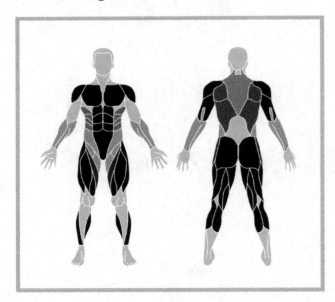

REBOOT

DAREBEE WORKOUT © darebee.com

LEVEL I 3 sets **LEVEL II** 5 sets **LEVEL III** 7 sets **REST** up to 2 minutes

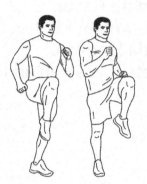 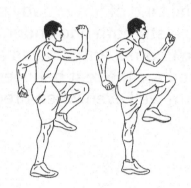 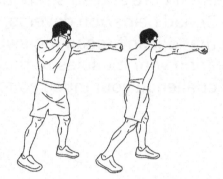

3combos: **20** high knees + **10** march   **40** punches

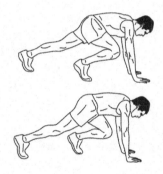 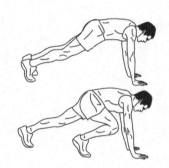 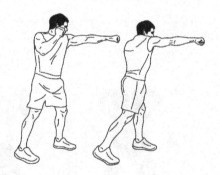

3combos: **20** climbers + **10** slow climbers   **40** punches

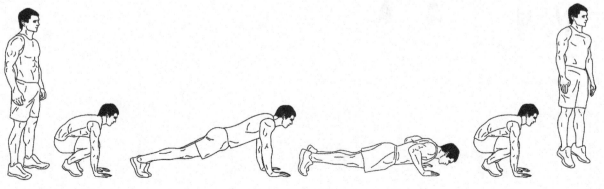

10 burpees (squat + plank + push-up + jump-in + jump up)

87 Recon Squad

To recon you need to be light on your feet, strong, agile and fast. You need great core and ab strength and the kind of lower body strength Recon Squad helps you develop. This is a strength and endurance workout but that doesn't mean the sweat won't come. It just takes a little longer to bring your muscles to the boil. Reduce the rest between sets if you can and challenge your muscles to perform well even when tired.

Focus: Strength & Tone

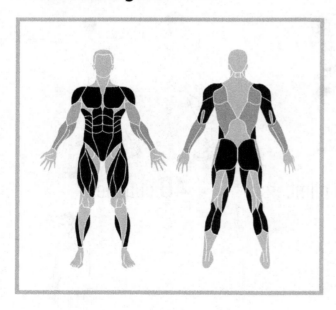

RECON SQUAD

DAREBEE WORKOUT
© darebee.com
LEVEL I 3 sets
LEVEL II 5 sets
LEVEL III 7 sets
REST up to 2 minutes

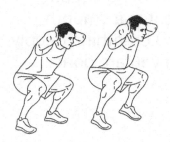

10 squat hops

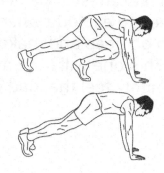

10 slow climbers

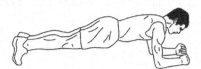

20-count elbow plank

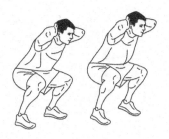

10 squat hops

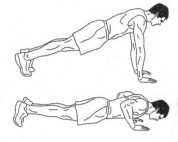

10 push-ups

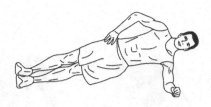

20-count side plank

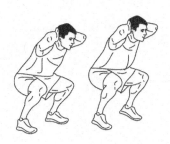

10 squat hops

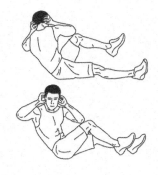

10 knee-to-elbows

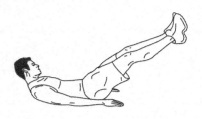

20-count raised leg hold

88 Recruit

Recruit is the workout that activates every muscle in your body and recruits several at a time to perform each exercise. The accent here is on form rather than speed. You don't need to explode when performing squats, for instance, but you do need to go deep and make sure it is a smooth, controlled motion throughout. This one will not have you breathing deeply at all but your muscles will definitely feel the load when you are done.

Focus: Strength & Tone

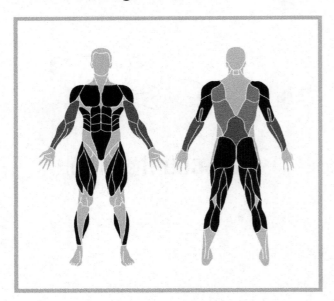

RECRUIT

DAREBEE WORKOUT © darebee.com

LEVEL I 3 sets **LEVEL II** 5 sets **LEVEL III** 7 sets **REST** up to 2 minutes

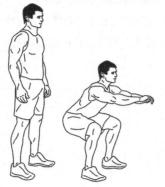

20 squats

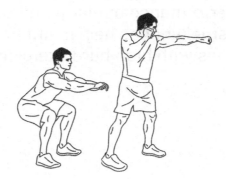

20 squat + jab

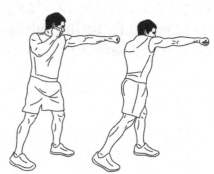

20 jab + cross

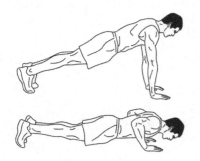

4 push-ups

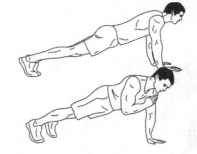

20 shoulder taps

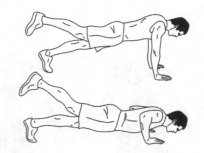

4 raised leg push-ups

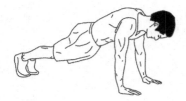

20-count plank

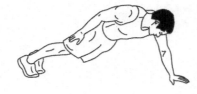

20-count one-arm plank

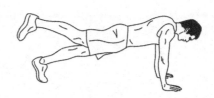

20-count raised leg plank

89 Scorcher

The Scorcher is a high burn full body workout that alternates the load from the muscles to the lungs and back again. Obviously all muscle activity requires good VO2 Max performance but larger muscle groups need more oxygen to function while smaller ones help maintain that familiar recover-on-the-fly feeling that comes with high-burn exercises.

Focus: High Burn

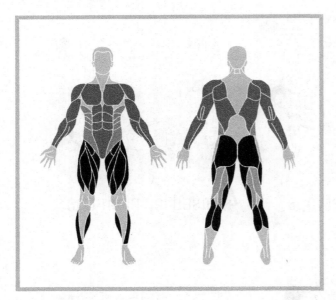

THE SCORCHER

DAREBEE CARDIO WORKOUT © darebee.com

LEVEL I 3 sets **LEVEL II** 5 sets **LEVEL III** 7 sets **REST** up to 2 minutes

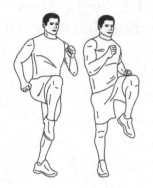

60 high knees

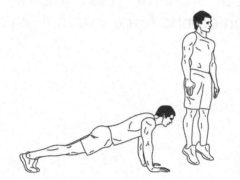

10 basic burpee w/ jump

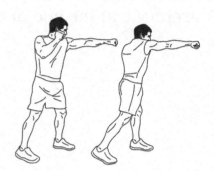

40 punches

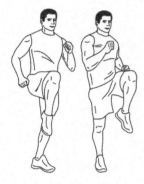

60 high knees

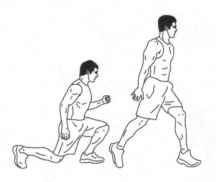

10 jumping lunges

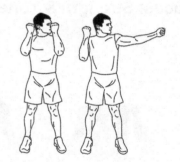

40 backfists

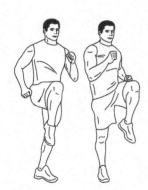

60 high knees

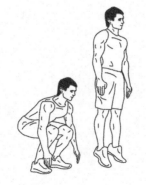

10 jump squats

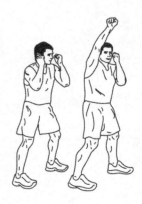

40 overhead punches

90 Sculptor

Sculpt your body, up your speed and push your aerobic performance to new heights with the Sculptor workout. This combines it all plus the slow exercises at the end of each combo force you to use your muscles fully.

Focus: Strength & Tone

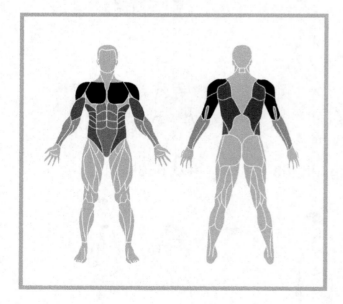

SCULPTOR

DAREBEE WORKOUT FOR ARMS, CHEST AND BACK
© darebee.com

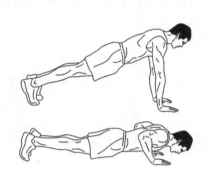
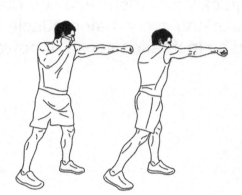

10 push-ups
40 punches
10 push-ups
40 punches
10 push-ups
40 punches
1 minutes rest

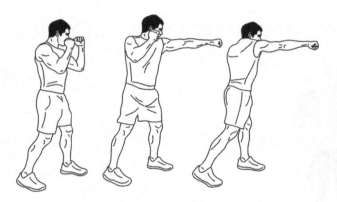

go as fast as you can, non-stop

1 minute punches
1 minutes rest
1 minute punches
1 minutes rest

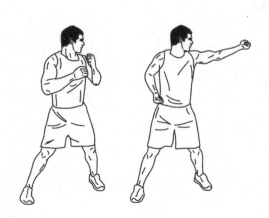

100 reps per side, then change.

200

backfists

Done!

Sentinel

Sentinel is a Level 4 total body strength workout. It's designed to push you into the sweat zone quickly and then keep you there as you go from one exercise to the next, working every major muscle group you have. It delivers strength, stability and an increased sense of power.

Focus: Strength & Tone

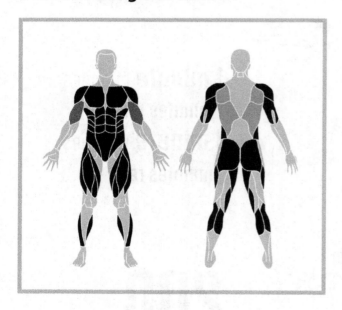

SENTINEL

DAREBEE WORKOUT © darebee.com

LEVEL I 3 sets **LEVEL II** 5 sets **LEVEL III** 7 sets **REST** up to 2 minutes

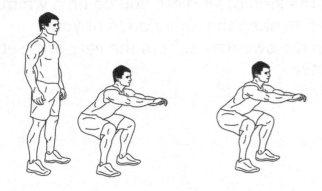

4combos: **10** squats + **10-count** hold

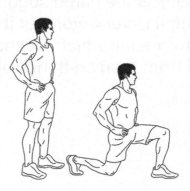

40 lunges

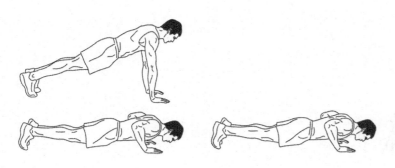

4combos: **5** push-ups + **5-count** hold

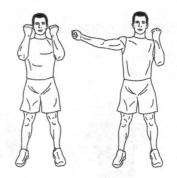

40 side-to-side backfists

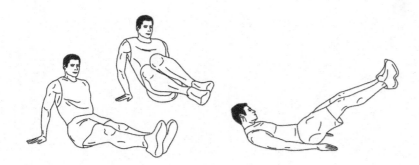

4combos: **10** knee-in & twist + **10-count** hold

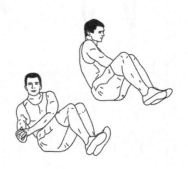

40 sitting twists

92   Sniper

Sniper, as the name suggests, is not the kind of workout you do on a whim. Being a Level 4 workout it is designed to push the boundaries of your performance which means you are in the sweatzone from the very first set and from then on things only get hotter.

Focus: Strength & Tone

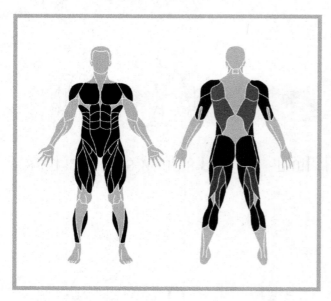

SNIPER

DAREBEE WORKOUT © darebee.com

LEVEL I 3 sets **LEVEL II** 5 sets **LEVEL III** 7 sets **REST** up to 2 minutes

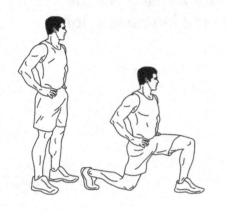
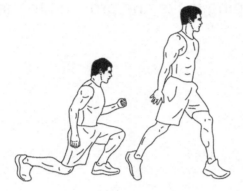
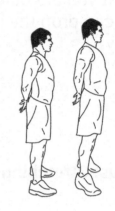

20 lunges   **20** jumping lunges   **20** calf raises

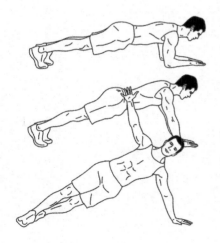
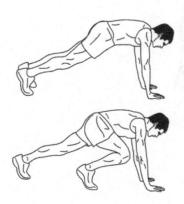
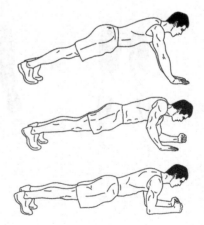

20 press w/ rotations   **20** climbers   **20** up & down planks

93 Splits

Doing the splits is a bucket-list thing for many. But here you can achieve that, in a gradual, step-by-step manner with the Splits workout. Make sure you maintain form throughout. Do it regularly.

Tip: If you are doing this routine post-workout (you are already warmed up) you can drop the jumping jacks and proceed to the side leg raises right away.

Focus: Stretching

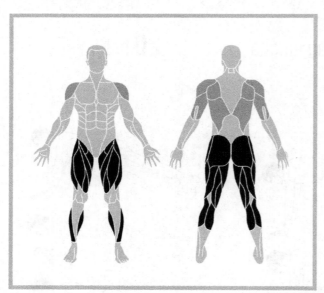

SPLITS

DAREBEE WORKOUT © darebee.com

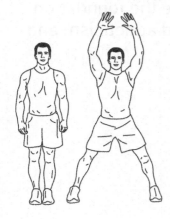

40 jumping jacks
1 minute rest
40 jumping jacks
1 minute rest
40 jumping jacks
1 minute rest

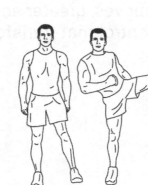

100 side leg raises

<u>Hold on to something</u> but
don't put your active
foot down. 50 raises per leg.

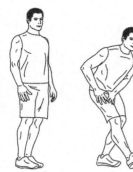
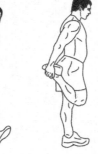
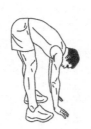

10 seconds each exercise; change legs
and do the exercise again on the other side

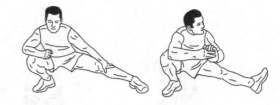

10 deep side-to-side lunges
10 deep side-to-side lunges toes up

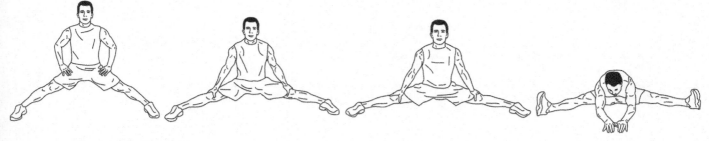

2 minutes side splits - go as low as you can, then sit down & lean forward
as illustrated above. Try to go further every time you do this workout.

94   Springboard

Springboard helps you work your quads, calves, glutes, lower tendons and abs and works hard to deliver fascial fitness. All of this are the foundation of building spring-like moves, greater endurance, improved athleticism and the kind of muscular control that transforms you entirely.

Focus: Strength & Tone

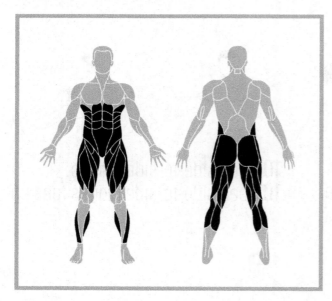

SPRINGBOARD

DAREBEE WORKOUT © darebee.com

LEVEL I 3 sets **LEVEL II** 5 sets **LEVEL III** 7 sets **REST** 2 minutes

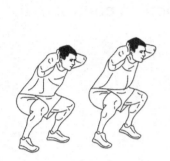

10 squat hops

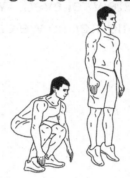

10 jump squats

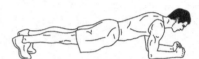

30sec elbow plank

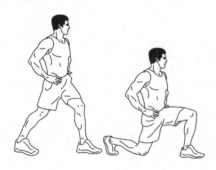

10 split lunges

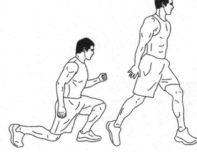

10 jumping lunges

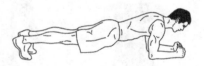

30sec elbow plank

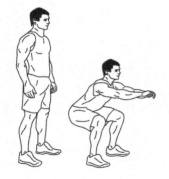

10 squats

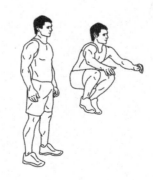

10 jump knee tucks

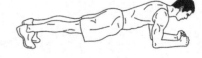

30sec elbow plank

95   Static Zap

When it comes to Level Five workouts Static Zap is designed to test your strength to the limit. From one exercise to the next muscle groups are loaded differently but not completely relieved. We always fight with our own body's weight. We want it to feel lighter so we can be more in control of it. Well, here's how that truly starts.

Focus: Strength & Tone

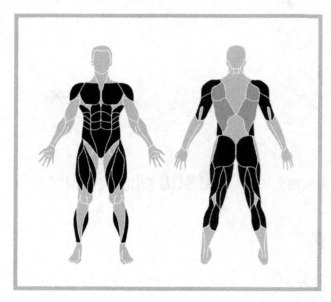

static zap

DAREBEE WORKOUT © darebee.com

LEVEL I 3 sets **LEVEL II** 5 sets **LEVEL III** 7 sets **REST** up to 2 minutes

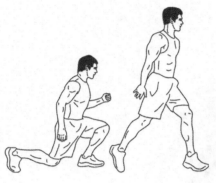

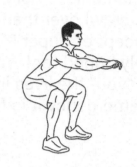

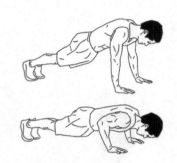

10-count push-up plank   **20** jumping lunges   **10-count** squat hold

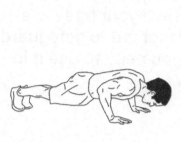

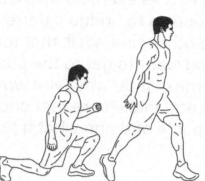

10-count push-up plank   **20** jumping lunges   **10** slow push-ups

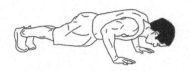

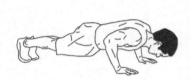

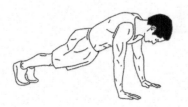

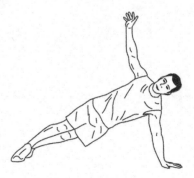

10-count push-up plank   **20-count** plank hold   **10-count** side plank

96 Super Plank

There is a Chinese Special Forces exercise where soldiers have to act as a human bridge, using their bodies to bridge a narrow chasm so their buddies can crawl over them to the other side. Well, that totally illustrates the concept of Super Plank. You want to get to the point where your body is a finely honed tool. You can make it do what you want. It is there to safeguard the "you" the lives inside it and make sure that should you need to use it in an emergency it is fully capable of doing what it has to.

Focus: Abs

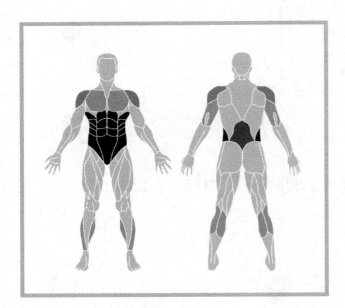

super plank

DAREBEE WORKOUT © darebee.com

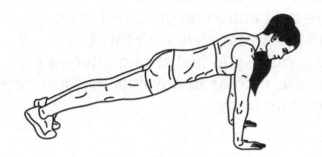

30sec plank

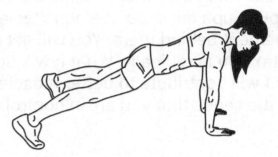

30sec wide leg plank

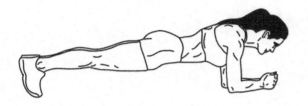

30sec elbow plank

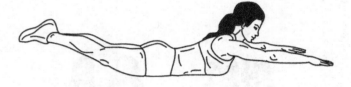

30sec superman plank

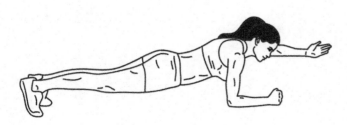

60sec raised arm elbow plank
30 seconds - each arm

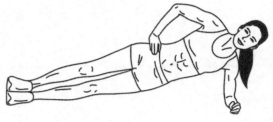

60sec side plank
30 seconds - each side

97 Tank Top

Tank Top is a strength workout that engages all upper body muscle groups and activates the core. This means the moves are slow and meticulous, the push ups are deep, the punches are deliberate and utilize a full body movement behind them. You will get in the sweat zone with this but it will not tax you aerobically. What it will do is make you feel strong afterwards and it will contribute to better muscle tone, increased physical performance and the sense that you are in control of your body.

Focus: Strength & Tone

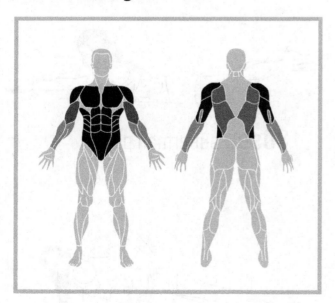

TANK TOP

DAREBEE WORKOUT
© darebee.com
LEVEL I 3 sets
LEVEL II 5 sets
LEVEL III 7 sets
REST up to 2 minutes

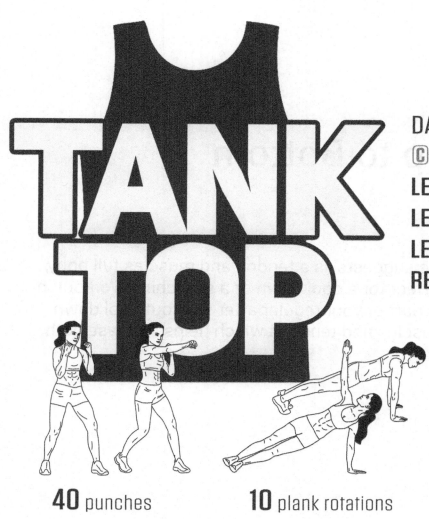

40 punches

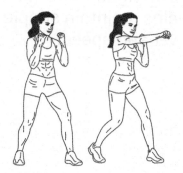

10 plank rotations

40 punches

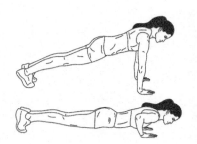

10 push-ups

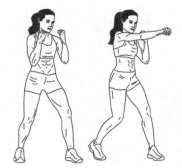

40 punches

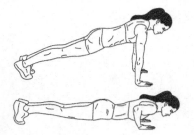

10 push-ups

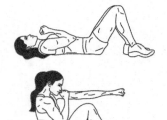

20 sit-up punches

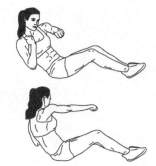

20 sitting punches

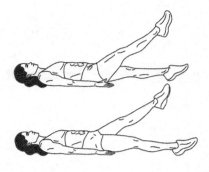

20 flutter kicks

Top to Bottom

Top To Bottom, as the name suggests, is a tendon and muscles full body, stretching routine that's perfect for a cool down or a stretching workout in its own right. Performed as part of your regular after-workout cool down it helps maintain supple muscles and tendons which helps increase both power and speed.

Focus: Stretching

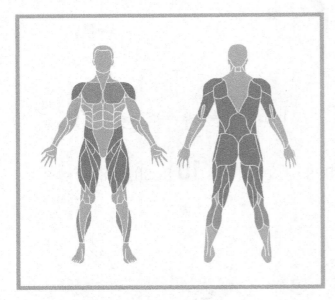

top to bottom

STRETCHING / COOLDOWN BY DAREBEE © darebee.com

Repeat each stretch for 20 seconds / 20 seconds per side.

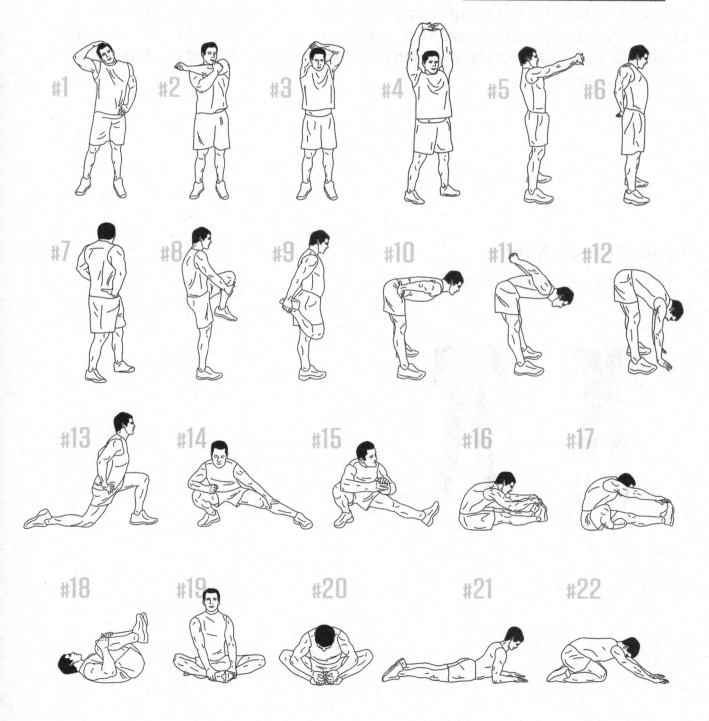

#1 #2 #3 #4 #5 #6

#7 #8 #9 #10 #11 #12

#13 #14 #15 #16 #17

#18 #19 #20 #21 #22

99 Valkyrie

Traditionally picked to choose who lived or died in battle Valkyries were warriors in the own right and warriors always need to have the capability to control their bodies and move fast, with grace, under pressure. The Valkyrie workout helps you develop the kind of strength, balance and muscle control that the role requires.

Focus: Strength & Tone

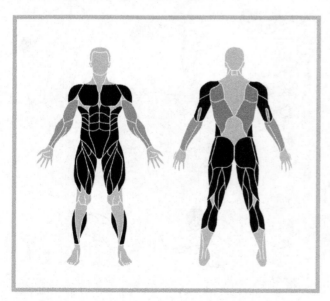

Valkyrìe

DAREBEE WORKOUT © darebee.com

LEVEL I 3 sets **LEVEL II** 5 sets **LEVEL III** 7 sets **REST** up to 2 minutes

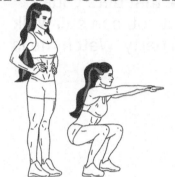

10 squats

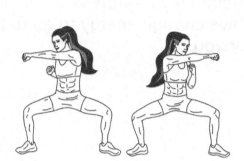

10 squat punches

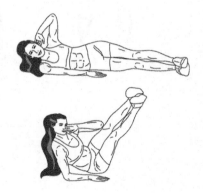

10 squat cross steps

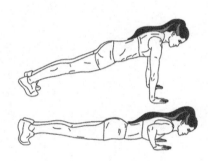

10 push-ups

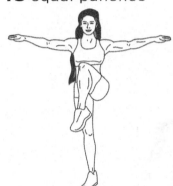

40sec balance stand

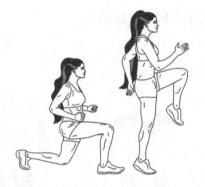

20 lunge step-ups

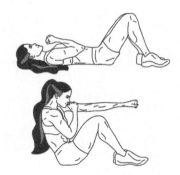

10 sit-up punches

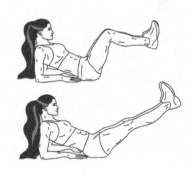

10 crunch kicks

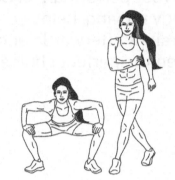

10 side Vs

100   Watch Me.

Not every full body workout need to try and push you to the very boundaries of your performance. Sometimes you need to have one that gets your body moving, helps you maintain your fitness levels but you can still walk straight afterwards and have enough energy to go to a party. Watch me is then the perfect choice for you.

Focus: High Burn

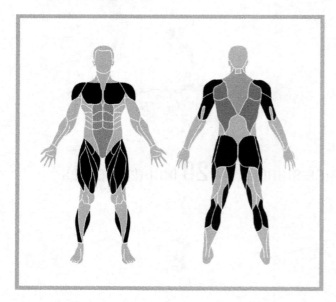

watch me.

DAREBEE CARDIO WORKOUT © darebee.com
LEVEL I 3 sets **LEVEL II** 5 sets **LEVEL III** 7 sets
REST up to 2 minutes

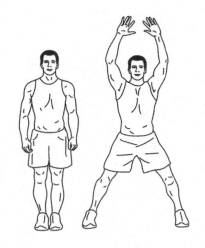

20 jumping jacks

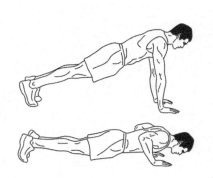

10 push-ups

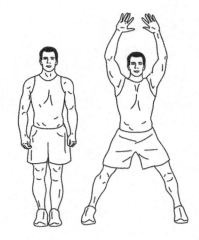

20 jumping jacks

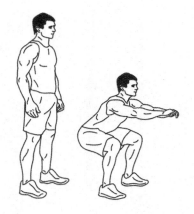

20 squats

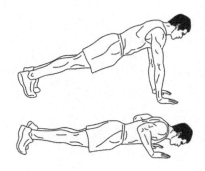

10 push-ups

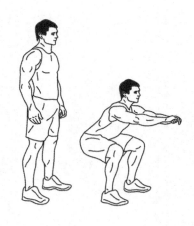

20 squats

Thank you!

Thank you for purchasing *100 No-Equipment Workouts*, Vol 2. DAREBEE project print edition. DAREBEE is a non-profit global fitness resource dedicated to making fitness accessible for everyone, no matter the circumstances. The project is supported exclusively via user donations and paperback royalties.

After printing cost and store fees every book developed by DAREBEE project makes $1 and it goes directly into our project maintenance and development fund.

Each sale helps us keep the DAREBEE resource growing, maintain it and keep it up. Thank you for making a difference in its future!